# Departure From the
# Darkness and the Cold

# Departure From the Darkness and the Cold

## The Hope of Renewal for the Soul of Medicine in Patient Care

**Lawrence J. Hergott, M.D.**

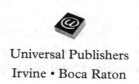

Universal Publishers
Irvine • Boca Raton

*Departure From the Darkness and the Cold:*
*The Hope of Renewal for the Soul of Medicine in Patient Care*

Universal Publishers, Inc.
Irvine • Boca Raton
USA • 2020
www.Universal-Publishers.com

ISBN: 978-1-62734-302-2 (pbk.)
ISBN: 978-1-62734-303-9 (ebk.)

Typeset by Medlar Publishing Solutions Pvt Ltd, India
Cover design by Ivan Popov

Library of Congress Cataloging-in-Publication Data

Names: Hergott, Lawrence J., 1946- author.
Title: Departure from the darkness and the cold : the hope of renewal for the soul of medicine in patient care / Lawrence J. Hergott, M.D.
Description: Irvine, California : Universal Publishers, Inc. 2020.
Identifiers: LCCN 2020004053 (print) | LCCN 2020004054 (ebook) | ISBN 9781627343022 (paperback) | ISBN 9781627343039 (ebook)
Subjects: LCSH: Medical care--Literary collections. | Physician and patient--Literary collections. Classification: LCC PS3608.E736 A6 2020 (print) | LCC PS3608.E736 (ebook) | DDC 808.8/03561--dc23
LC record available at https://lccn.loc.gov/2020004053
LC ebook record available at https://lccn.loc.gov/2020004054

*For Sienna,*

*And a Life of Love*

# TABLE OF CONTENTS

# ACKNOWLEDGEMENTS

## Most Grateful For
My beloved sweetheart, sage, listener, laugher, best friend, and mother of our children—Diane Bachaus Hergott, with whom I fell in love in September 1963.

My loving children Matthew, Leah, and Zachary—all of whom have generated pride and awe in me.

My granddaughter, Sienna, to whom this book is dedicated, and her father, Tom, who is a marvelous husband, father, and son-in-law.

## In Medicine
Dr. Ezra Amsterdam, who believed in me as a cardiologist and person during my training and beyond.

Dr. James Rogers Fox, who when I was a teenager enchanted me about medicine from his weekday 15-minute afternoon television program in Minneapolis.

Dr. Philip Wolf, whose enthusiasm for my first essay lead me to a university position and here.

## In Writing
Many of whom impassioned in me what Alan Bennett expressed to a student in his play, *The History Boys*:

> "The best moments in reading...are when you come across something—a thought...a feeling...a way of looking at things—that you'd thought special...particular to you—and here it is! Set down by someone else...a person you've never met...maybe even someone long dead. And...it's as if a hand has come out... and taken yours."

Buckminster Fuller, who opened the world—scientifically and immortally—to me.

John O'Donohue, a graciously loving, brilliant, down to Earth Irish philosopher and writer from West-of-Ireland farmland who left us too soon.

Roger Rosenblatt, whose wisdom, writing, and generosity I came across years ago, and benefit from still.

Dr. Michael LaCombe, cardiologist, sage, and editor of *Annals of Internal Medicine*, whose guidance has enhanced my writing.

Dr. Jack Coulehan, everyone's *emeritus writer of medicine*, who has kindly taken the time and effort to write the foreward in this book.

David Whyte, whose book, *The Heart Aroused*, was the source of interest that ignited my writing.

Roxanne K. Young, a former editor of the *Journal of the American Medical Association* (*JAMA*) who at first nurtured and then supported my essays in *JAMA*.

Don Talafous, O.S.B., a Benedictine monk who has been a friend and exemplar since my first year in college.

Dr. Martina Schulte, physician and coach specializing in individuals and organizations dealing with professional satisfaction and burnout—who has worked diligently to review this book's manuscript, and offer sage advice.

Dr. John Harper, whose everlasting efforts to broaden medical prose and poetry is a gift renowned.

Kay and Matthew Bucksbaum, who benevolently encouraged my writing from the first time they read it in a hospital room.

Thomas Friedman, whose wide-ranging, profound, and soulful writing in the *New York Times* and his books not only enlightens readers but enhances their compassion.

Sisters Mary Luke Tobin and Cecily Jones, beloved *Sisters of Loretto*, who when in Kentucky were friends of Thomas Merton—and who in a nondenominational book club in Denver years ago beneficently introduced me to Merton and themselves.

Thomas Merton, Trappist monk, mystic, author, and more, whose brilliance, depth, and courage in writing enhances mine—and my own sense of self.

Jeff Young at Universal Publishers for his guidance and encouragement.

# FOREWORD

Sometime in the early 1980s, I fell into a mid-life crisis. I had a loving wife, a growing family, considerable academic success, and a great deal of satisfaction taking care of patients. So what could be lacking? Seamus Heaney's translation of the opening lines of Dante's *Inferno* almost exactly captured my predicament:

> In the middle of the journey of our life
> I found myself astray in a dark wood
> where the straight road had been lost sight of.
>
> How hard it is to say what it was like
> in the thicket of thickets, in a wood so dense and gnarled
> the very thought of it renews my panic.[1]

After some struggle, I found that my straight road forward lay in poetry. I began to write. Well, it wasn't the poetry itself that freed me from the thicket, but rather the process of reflection and self-discovery that resulted in poems. It turned out that the meaning in my life had been present all around me. I just hadn't fully experienced it. As William Osler wrote, "Nothing will sustain you more potently in your humdrum routine...than the power to recognize the true poetry of life—the poetry of the commonplace, of the ordinary man, of the plain, toil-worn woman, with their loves and their joys, their sorrows and their griefs."[2]

In this wonderful collection of essays and poems, Lawrence Hergott employs Dante's "lost in a dark wood" as a metaphor to today's physicians and the profession as a whole. These are difficult times. Multiple external pressures threaten the core values of medicine—empathy, compassion, excellence, fidelity, integrity, and humility. Many physicians are sensing that indeed the right road has been lost sight of. They ask themselves how to pursue a life of service in a world of markets and machines? How to maintain a healing bond with patients in the era of Big Medicine? What is happening to the soul of medicine?

Dr. Hergott addresses these questions with experience and insight. A veteran of decades of medical practice, he witnesses to the burden and sacrifice, as well as the profound personal fulfillment, of a life in medicine. He acknowledges external pressures but, in his stories and reflections, he serves as a role model of resilience and creativity, suggesting how others, young physicians and medical students, might discover their own straight road.

These are the reflections of a thoughtful physician about his life experience as a whole, not just tales of treating patients. We learn of Dr. Hergott's great personal loss, the death of his son in an airplane crash, but also about the quiet joy he and his wife experienced when his career change offered the prospect of spending more time with family. We read of his "Blessing for a Newborn Child," and mull over his poem of gratitude, "A Letter to a Dying Friend." A full life, and a full experience for the reader.

In one of his essays, Dr. Hergott quotes Joseph Campbell as saying, "The trouble we are having in the United States, doctors, is that we are often practicing medicine as *prose* rather than the *poetry* it really is."

Lawrence Hergott practices as poetry.
Jack Coulehan, MD, MPH

# References

1.  Heaney S. Canto One. In *Dante's Inferno*, New York, Daniel Halpern (Ed.) The Ecco Press, 1993, p. 3.
2.  Osler W. The student life. In *Osler's 'A Way of Life' & Other Addresses With Commentary & Annotations*, Eds. S Hinohara and H Niki, Durham, Duke University Press, 2001, p. 305.

# INTRODUCTION

I am writing the beginning of this introduction sitting in a cloistered square enclosed by the stone walls of a hospital Queen Isabella and King Ferdinand built in the Spanish town of Santiago de Compostela in 1501. The long wooden table I write on is more than 150 years old, as is the small but exceedingly heavy wooden chair on which I sit. The center of the square is filled with a sculpted, arched stone well, waist-high deep-green bushes, and a vast assortment of pleasurably colored flowers brightened by a radiant sun. The square is a meditative, inspirational place in which to contemplate and write.

When Isabella and Ferdinand came to visit Santiago de Compostela, they were troubled by the mutilation of many of the pilgrims who walked, sometimes hundreds of miles—"poorly fed and uncleansed"—to get to the Santiago de Compostela Cathedral to pray for help from St. James, one of Jesus' apostles. Legend has it that the cathedral contains the bones of St. James, and pilgrims have journeyed to the cathedral for over a thousand years to seek his help. Pilgrims who arrived unwell could be treated at the ancient hospital at no charge and for as long as it took to restore their health.

I decided to write in the square not only because it is pleasant to be here, but also because it imparts a sense of depth to ponder disturbing inconsistencies between what the ancient hospital symbolized and accomplished long ago, and the structure of medical practice today that does the opposite, and imperils the wellbeing of both patients and physicians. *Departure From the Darkness and the Cold: The Hope of Renewal for the Soul of Medicine in Patient Care* is written in the spirit of hope that this transgression will be undone. An explanation of how and what has transgressed follows, which will set the stage for the stories and poems in the content of the book, which serve to encourage clinicians—physicians, physicians' assistants, nurse practitioners, nurses, pharmacists, etc.—to persevere. An explanation of the transgressions can also help non-medical readers understand the dilemma, and also get a glimpse of *the life of medicine* today.

The major force of this misdirected situation is the loss of freedom for physicians in the current era, who now lead torturously intense and dispiritingly long days appeasing business-based overlords rather than giving comprehensive care to patients. One major miscalculation that affects clinicians' clinic and hospital days is that they are now forced to regularly perform trivial, superfluous acts, similar to what John Muir described as "*cold enslaving musts*"—the experience that motivated him to escape from his job as a woodcutter to fulfill his passion for nature, thus giving his gift to the world.

At least at present, the great majority of clinicians, though in various states of duress, continue to work diligently to honor the call of caring they devoted themselves to, and remain true to what the late Irish philosopher and poet John O'Donohue offered in his poem, *For Presence*, "Respond to the call of your gift and the courage to follow its path."

Tragically, an increasing number of clinicians are following Muir's course, and literally escaping from their jobs. *How* medical practice changed and led to this harmful and non-sustaining state is well defined. Since *what* has risen from the changes is more relevant to this book than *how* the dysfunction occurred, I will offer an extensive description of the *what*, but start by briefly summarizing the *how*.

The source of sorrow—and anger—clinicians have carried in recent years relates to the mismanagement of challenges in contemporary medicine that were inconceivable a few decades ago. Decisions were made from these challenges mostly by nonclinical administrators—business oriented healthcare organizations, insurance companies, hospital executives, etc. Actions largely focused on productivity and profit rather than the foundational, healing practices of quality and concern, have thus overtaken the structure of patient care, and relegated clinicians to the level of pawns rather than highly valued individuals dedicated to the welfare of others. In centering on the business aspects of the structure of medical delivery, healthcare leaders and executives have violated a proverb Buckminster Fuller declared in his book, *Critical Path*—a statement relevant to many modes of service, and certainly to medical practice—"You can make money, or you can make sense." Also violated is Sir William Osler's elucidation over a century ago of what medicine was, and is: "The practice of medicine is an art, not a trade; a calling, not a business; a calling in which your heart will be exercised equally with your head."

Physicians bear some responsibility for our current race to the bottom as well. We may not have paid enough attention, for example, to the rising and excessive costs of clinical care prior to the changes mentioned, or of our role in lowering those costs. Some physicians have tragically put their own monetary benefit ahead of patients' needs— doing more procedures, operations, and interventions for profit rather than healing. As mentioned in the essay, *The View From Fiesole*, I asked a physician who called me to see if he could join our university group just why he wanted to join us. He said, "You know, to make it in the private world these days you have to sell your soul"—a statement bad enough on its own, but made even more troubling by his adding, "and I'm not sure I want to do that."

Regarding *what* has changed for the worse, many scientific papers— including those championed by Drs. Mark Linzer, Tait Shanafelt, Christine Sinsky, and others—describe medical practitioners' dissatisfaction in the current era. Data from the Emory University 2017–2018 Blue Ridge Academic Health Group summary paper indicate that about 54% of active physicians are not only unhappy but "burned out" in their work. In some specialties burnout may be as much as 70%. Those in the higher percentages are clinicians who are at the frontline of care—emergency room physicians, family medicine doctors, and internal medicine physicians especially. Aware of this, fewer medical students are showing interest in primary care careers, which are increasingly felt to be challenging and unsustainable. Also at the higher percentages of burnout are young and female doctors. In a 2019 *New England Journal of Medicine* article a national survey of general surgery residents demonstrated that mistreatment (discrimination, verbal or physical abuse, and sexual harassment) occurred frequently among the residents—especially in women—and is associated with burnout and suicidal thoughts. This finding is of exceptional importance because suicide is the second leading cause of death among trainees.

Elements of physician burnout listed in various studies include: less time with patients and the ability to nurture caring relationships; an erosion of the sense of meaning or fulfillment in medical practice; the possibility of decreased physical empathy for patients; a growing incidence of medical errors; loss of work-life balance, including inadequate time for families and intimate relationships, inadequate sleep, an often unbalanced diet, and absent exercise regimens; a growing rate of physicians leaving their practice (i.e., a 'turnover', the lost revenue of one person leaving a group being $500,000 or more); and, an increase in "pajama time"—spending late evenings at home doing catchup work on a computer, at the expense of rest and relaxation, and even professional literature review.

A research paper headed by Dr. Sinsky showed that in an ambulatory clinic setting physicians spent nearly two hours on desk and electronic medical record duties for every hour spent face-to-face with a patient.

A study from the American Medical Group Association (AMGA) shows that the rate of early retirement has increased from 12% to 18%.

A friend planning early retirement summarized our current troubles well: "It is becoming more and more difficult trying to keep up. The workload keeps increasing without a concomitant increase in technical and professional manpower support—doing more with less, for less, and faster, seems to be the thinking of administration."

It is because of *what* has happened to clinicians from imperiling changes that *Departure From the Darkness and the Cold: The Hope of Renewal for the Soul of Medicine in Patient Care* is written. Because of the troubles described, the spirit-killing sense so many physicians carry have left an integral and transcendent part of patient care, the *soul of medicine*, smoldering in the distance rather than blazing within us. I define the soul of medicine as: *That thing beyond the biomedical, immutable, and sustaining: the caring, compassionate, dedicated, enthusiastic attitude that set us on the difficult-by-nature, enriching journey called the medical life.* Medical practitioners yearn to rekindle the soul of medicine, and be fully present and helpful to patients again.

With the epidemic we face being well defined and devolving, attempts to correct the course we are on have begun. Various universities, practices, and healthcare organizations are attempting to adopt wellness agendas, and are beginning to lay out ways to minimize the physical, intellectual, and emotional stresses of healthcare personnel—to the benefit of not only clinicians, but patients and healthcare organizations as well. Our long and complicated first pass at offering modern-day medical care has failed. Achieving our goal will require a broader perspective than before, and cooperation rather than seclusion in the people involved. Parties developing our reconstruction, together, could benefit from reflecting on the fact that Daedalus did not tell Icarus to keep from flying too close to the sun. He ordered Icarus to fly the middle course, and avoid not only the heat of the sun but the spray of the sea, which could bring him down. Our first try at the delivery of contemporary health care avoided flying too close to the sun, but crashed by being brought down from the unknown risk of the ocean spray.

Working together, all of us learning from our mistakes, and dedicated to the benefit of others more than ourselves, we can create a lifegiving and honorable system. It is in hope that such an alliance will pronounce as its foundation a quote from the Chinese sage, Chuang Tzu: *'When the heart is right, For and Against are forgotten.'*

A statement from Dr. Donald M. Berwick, of the Institute for Healthcare Improvement, offers a view of who we are and what we are as clinicians, and where we should be heading:

"It has long seemed a paradox to me that such depletion of joy in work can pervade as noble and meaningful an enterprise as health care. What we in the healing professions and its support roles get to do every day touches the highest aspirations of a compassionate civilization. We have chosen a calling that invites people who are worried and suffering to share their stories and allow us to help. If any work ought to give spiritual satisfaction to the workers, this is it. 'Joy,' not 'burnout,' ought to rule the day."

Until that day comes, we will need inspiration and hope if we are to sustain. The stories and poems in this book manifest acts in which the soul of medicine is not only present but flaming, stories and poems intended to remind experienced clinicians of when there was *time for kindness*, and, so different from now, how good it felt to treat patients in a caring, enthusiastic, unfettered way—a time when medical practice could feel nothing short of joyful. The sharing of stories and poems can also serve as encouragement for medical trainees and those considering a life in medicine, fostering hope that in their practice they will experience the kinds of interactions that used to be common.

Beyond the importance of adjusting medical practice so that doctors can flourish and deliver comprehensive care lies a more global need—the restitution of the field of medicine itself. As mentioned in the essay, *Lost in a Dark Wood*, think about what happens to a society when its most educated and humanistic individuals function as frenetic technicians in creativity killing systems. Think about what a culture loses when people with admirable traits work so intensely on assigned tasks that little energy is left for anything except (perhaps) an insular existence focused on one's immediate family. There is much for doctors to attend to beyond their practice, and they need time and effort to do so. It might not be an overstatement to say that at this time, as stated in *Lost in a Dark Wood*, the *true way* is *wholly lost*.

Doctors have always provided a voice on behalf of humanity. It is critical now for physicians to expand their relevance and dedication to life, and speak out about the physical and mental dangers from global warming, gun violence, universal epidemics, nuclear weapons, etc. Think about what future generations of physicians, society, and the world will be like if we do not return to the *true way*.

--------

In addition to what medical practitioners might take from reading this book, the stories and poems are also directed toward general public readers, so they can better understand how their doctors lead the fascinating and enigmatic medical life—and how that life may affect themselves as patients. The stories told and poems offered *lift the veil* that shades the medical life, and allows nonmedical readers to perceive many of its aspects. While there is a foundation of science in the telling of the stories and poems this is not a scientific book. What is mostly described are interactions between medical personnel and patients that can be understood by nonmedical readers, especially as they recognize the presence of the soul of medicine in the interactions. As John O'Donohue declared about writing, "You respect the dignity and potential of the reader." Considering the complexity and depth of medicine, without an entrance such as the book, patients and their loved ones can know very little about their doctors.

A striking example of the disparity between what a patient might perceive in an office or hospital visit and what a doctor brings into the room begins with a question my father-in-law asked of me regarding medicine: "Well, it's mostly just visiting isn't it?" The details of that question and its answer are in the chapter, *Alvin*. The disparities of my father-in-law's perception and what his family doctor brought into the room is nothing short of gargantuan, as the chapter reveals. There is much that is wondrous under the veil.

The essays and poems you will read are actual events people in the medical family have experienced. What is written is intended to offer interesting—and profound, and heartfelt, and sometimes humorous—encounters they have met.

The first essay in the book, *The Time of the Three Dynasties*, describes the troubles doctors and their loved ones experienced in the 1990's, before the radical changes in medicine added to our difficulties. The title of the essay comes from the ancient Chinese philosopher, Chuang Tzu—a salient question that applies to doctor's now:

*From the time of the Three Dynasties men have been running in all directions. How can they find time to be human?*

The beginning of the essay tells the story of the death of my brother-in-law in a farm accident, and my realizing when our family went back to our small hometown to stay with his family that in essence the stresses he felt were much like those of physicians. Several stories are told about specific troubles physicians endured—and a few examples of some doctors making lifegiving changes upon their understanding the threatening implications of their troubles.

The poem, *A Small, Sacred Space*, expresses the clarity and comfort a doctor offers to a physician-friend anticipating the dangerous removal of a brain tumor.

The essay, *The Desktop Photo*, describes a critical decision a cardiothoracic surgeon had to face between medicine and his family. Medical practice can easily cause imbalance between its needs and a doctor's family—and too often leads to what Frank Lloyd Wright said about himself not being a good family man, "The architect absorbed the father."

*A Tender, Comforting Something* is a poem about a physician who is fretful over the troubles of people unknown and far away. His apprehension manifests the broad relevance of concern that doctors can have even for strangers, the presence of the soul of medicine as their base. The poem is dedicated with gratitude to *New York Times* columnist Thomas Friedman, whose work over decades has demonstrated such concern for such people.

The poem, *A Separate Sacrifice*, offers what, how, and why a medical family can endure when a physician is on duty and absent.

*An Elevator Blessing* is an essay that demonstrates, in a descent in an elevator, how doctors can be of soulful benefit to patients not even their own, and in the most common of circumstances.

The poem, *Tragedy of Shadows*, given the 2015 *Annals Poetry Prize*—awarded by the international medical journal, *Annals of Internal Medicine*—depicts the shrouded "why" of the loss of a physician's beloved.

A particularly poignant essay, *A Single Cloud Eclipses the Sun*, begins with a moment-to-moment description of a tragic, erroneous outcome from a decision I made on a patient in my first year as a cardiologist. The essay goes on to describe what clinicians may carry forever when even a single judgment that harms one patient is made.

The next essay, *Facing Our Mistakes*, goes into detail about how hard clinicians work to avoid harming patients, dedicated always to the tenet, *primum non nocere—first do no harm*. The essay also shares some of the responsibilities physicians carry, and how they might progress over time when harm is done, to recover enough to persist in their call to heal—enough of a recovery to enter the room where the next patient sits, waiting in anticipation. The essay describes ways to approach recovery, including such things as following the sayings of sages from Chuang Tzu to Thomas Merton.

The essay, *Playing the Moonlight Sonata From Memory*, is a passionate call for awareness of the wonders of medicine in physicians, which present themselves in our work hour after hour, day after day. Missing out or passing by such wonders is easy and understandable as we move through our intense and complex lives. The stories told in the essay serve for doctors to feel and appreciate the benefits available to them by moving beyond the biomedical, physical aspects of patient care, and considering the medical life in its whole.

The poem, *Sala de Esperanza*, considers the feelings and significance of loved ones as they sit in a waiting room anticipating the outcome of their beloved's treatment.

The poignant essay, *What She Saw*, affirms the profoundly deep connection that can occur between patients and their doctors—even when physically impossible.

The most personal of my experiences mentioned in the book begins with the essay, *A Journey Beyond Imagining*, which describes our family losing a son and brother with the death of our beloved Zachary in a plane crash. The theme of the essay describes experiences of myself and others in my going back to work after Zach's death. The essay not only describes my feelings in the months after returning to work, but also offers stories of many colleagues, friends, and even people I didn't know who helped sustain me—many of whom shared their experiences of loss as well. The essay also shares our family's learning, over time, to attain, "Freedom from the tyranny of grief in the midst of grief," as theological writer and clinical psychologist James Finley attests about grief and a number of other calamitous happenings.

The poem, *The Teardrop Approach*, is about Zach's death as well, but also addresses others who have not had a loss. *A Journey Beyond Imagining* and *The Teardrop Approach* were published in two international medical journals, The *Journal of the American Medical Association* (*JAMA*), and *Annals of Internal Medicine*, the same week, Thanksgiving Week in 2009, so that some medical families gathered together that week might benefit from them.

An example of such families doing so is a poignant email sent to me by an internist and mother of two sons, the email's title being, "I want you to know I have stopped cleaning my house." She related that she was "madly" cleaning her house in anticipation of a large gathering there on Thanksgiving Day. Noticing some unread journals that had to be cleared, she picked up an issue of *JAMA* and read *A Journey Beyond Imagining*. "Then I read it again," she wrote. "I turned to *Annals* and read *Teardrop Approach*. I just wanted you to know that I have stopped cleaning my house and am going to sit on the couch with my sons and just hold them, whether they like it or not."

A second response to the essay was that of the father of a *JAMA* subscriber writing to say that his daughter had him read it when he was at her house at Thanksgiving. He found it "almost impossible to read because I was still brushing away tears when my daughter's guests arrived." A number of people expressed being tearful while reading the essay and poem, another sign of their usefulness, I think. Many of the tears were clearly in sympathy for my family. Others, of course, had much to do with the readers' lives.

*A Journey Beyond Imagining* and *The Teardrop Approach* are followed later in the book by the essay, *The Absence of Something*, and the poem, *Some Years Having Passed Since I Lost You*, all being initiated by Zachary's death but relevant to many readers. Our family's story of loss is no more worthy of the telling than any family's. The essays and poems about Zachary's death were not written so readers could understand what happened to us. They are written for the benefit of others— those who have experienced loss, and those who have not.

The essay, *Contemplating the Loss of the Last GI*, begins with a patient in a Coronary Care Unit having chest pain. The history taken by the cardiologist included the source and importance of his chest pain, which was benign, as well as his previous health and social history. These lead to the knowledge of the patient's having been a soldier in WWII. The story expands to the cardiologist's interviewing WWII veterans across Colorado, a visit to see other veterans at a graduation ceremony in New Hampshire, a trip to Omaha Beach in Normandy, and a return to the Coronary Care Unit, where another WWII veteran lay dying from a severe heart valve malfunction.

The context of the essay is replete with the soul of medicine from the beginning, and also filled with stories of honor, gratitude, courage, belonging, and humility.

*What I Learned From John Denver* is an essay about how music and an artist's wisdom and sincerity helped in the evolution of a struggling physician-in-training—and in his life personally.

Dozens more essays and poems share scenes of medical practitioner-patient interactions that manifest the *soul of medicine*.

-------

It took a long time and much effort to write this book. While doing so, I was often reminded of something Jean Cocteau declared about creativity: "The muses don't invite you in. They open the door and point to the tightrope." Still, writing the book was a pleasure, largely because of the good fortune one has in doing so of sharing tales about the wonders of medicine and the wondrous people who live it.

Thank you for joining me on this literary journey. I hope you find some wisdom and light in our time together—and have a pleasant time doing so.

-- LJH --

# PROLOGUE

We begin with the essay, *Galileo's Grapes*, the theme of which is gratitude. The essay was written mostly in thanks for the many medical colleagues I have had the honor to work with over a long career. What is written, though, could apply to many people, medical or not, who fit the description of grace, virtue, and other praiseworthy traits mentioned in the essay. Someone you know may fit the description, and perhaps awaken the gratitude you have for that person. Perhaps the characteristics in the essay fit you. If so, I would encourage you to recognize and claim that designation, and take the time to ponder the experiences and meaning that brought you to it.

You may find someone or yourself as well in other essays and poems in this book—each of which originates from actions individuals have taken, but which has meaning for a much broader gathering in this celebration of charity and goodness.

-------

# GALILEO'S GRAPES

*The sun, with all those planets revolving around it ... can
still ripen a bunch of grapes as if it had nothing else in the
universe to do.*

– Galileo Galilei

Not one given to visions, I still feel as if I actually saw them, there on
the deck as I swam at the old Fitzsimons Army Hospital pool in Colorado. They were young men, their bodies pale, translucent, and incomplete. Each had part of an arm or a leg missing or had some other
wound inconsistent with the perfection of the rest of the body. They
were World War II GIs recuperating in the 1940s from battle injuries,
as so many veterans at Fitzsimons had before the base was recently
decommissioned. Most of them sat on a long wooden bench, silently
gazing at the water's reflection. A few moved clumsily for short dis-
tances along the deck, some embarrassed by their awkwardness, others
visibly frustrated. As I swam I wondered what it had been like for them
to be there and what had happened to them after they left. I felt very
sorry about what had happened to them in war and deeply grateful for
what they had done for me, unborn, so long ago. Then, they were gone,
at least from sight.

Having seen WW II veterans as patients virtually every day of my
career, I began reflecting more deeply about them only a few years ago.
The "vision" at the pool reminded me of my gratitude toward them
and has made me think more about gratitude in general. One of the
benefits of having had a long career is there being much to look back
on. A disadvantage is that so much has happened, a lot is forgotten.
I know, however, that for all of the individual effort required over four

decades of training and practice, I did not get to this point on my own. I have benefited from the mostly caring and supportive environment intrinsic to medicine. As opposed to some other professions that are inherently competitive or even adversarial, medicine is collaborative and strongly net positive rather than zero sum. While it would be an overstatement to say that every coworker we see during the workday is motivated primarily by altruism, I have been struck in noting that, effectively, the work each person does is for the benefit of someone else. Ultimately, we show up to help patients, their loved ones, and each other. Like Galileo's grapes, the medical family inhabits a grand system that is essentially sustaining and nurturing.

Thinking about things like gratitude takes quiet time, something medical practitioners and others have less of these days. Even the inclination to ponder such things is reduced with the contraction of physicians' interests in the past decade from the effect of practice constraints imposed on us. Having experienced these pressures intensely myself, I can readily confirm the truth of Baltasar Gracian's statement from the 17th century that "Life is painful without a rest." I would add that life without a rest can also be life unexamined or, worse, unnoticed. I can think of few things more unnatural or less acceptable to the practice of medicine. Ours is by nature an intense and vivid work, full of wonder and meaning. These properties are immutable even if our appreciation of them may fade over time. Although its form has changed, medicine continues to deliver on its promise to be the grand work it seemed when we were first drawn to it. I believe that the great majority of physicians come to medicine because of a love of science and a desire to help others. We subject ourselves to the field's arduous training and practice because we see a role for us in relation to the principle that, as Ian McEwan stated in his book Atonement, "A person is, among all else, a material thing, easily torn, not easily mended." I am frequently reminded of how useful we are to others even in the most elemental work we perform. How else to explain the depth of joy and tenderness I saw last week as a young couple quietly reached for each other after I told them that the woman's newly diagnosed congenital heart defect should have no bearing on her pregnancy. They think I made their day. They certainly made mine.

As in life generally, not everyone or everything we have experienced in medicine has been pleasant or helpful. But the great preponderance has been. In fact, there is so much that is good, one has to work to recall some of it. I can identify people and institutions spanning the entire period from well before the beginning of my medical education to the present to whom I am grateful. Some contributed directly to the colossal expansion of factual knowledge common to every physician's experience. Others played supportive or nurturing roles or simply made life interesting along the way.

Returning to academe in the last third of my career, I have experienced a renewed appreciation for physicians-in-training. I have the opportunity to interact with them at every phase of their medical education, from those just in off the street in their first weeks of medical school to others like our senior cardiothoracic surgery fellows in postgraduate year fourteen, superbly trained and ready now to return to serve the society they came from. The transformation I see in these young people is breathtaking. I am especially gratified to report that even with the social benefits many physicians-in-training have had over those of previous generations, their dedication and work ethic seem no less than those of their forebears. I am convinced, too, that their personal effort is the only thing that exceeds the help they get along the way and that without ample amounts of both they would not succeed. Adding to the knowledge of their transformation an understanding of what physicians in practice go through has persuaded me that no matter what specific direction it takes, the course of a medical life is nothing short of astonishing—a rich example of those Ernest Hemingway described as living life "full up."

Remarkable for me too is gratitude for physicians of times past, whose factual knowledge and therapeutic tools may have been comparatively limited but whose dedication and perseverance were not. I recall outstanding teachers, role models, and fellow house officers I had who in those formative years affirmed an inexperienced and often unconfident young physician. Later came talented practice partners whose commitment to patients and each other only deepened as medical practice devolved over the years. I am grateful to medical researchers and those who fund them for providing treatments that are common now but that could only be wished for earlier in my career.

Throughout I have benefited from a loving family, affirming patients and staffs, and, everywhere I have worked, nurses whose devotion to those in their care has been nothing short of inspirational. I have been greatly heartened, too, by the work of those who create or present music, art, and literature.

How about you? Who or what has inspired you? Given you confidence? Sustained you? Treated you with respect no matter what category you occupied at the time? Reassured you? Been loyal? Given you hope? Been gentle with you? Been hard on you when necessary? Made you laugh? Stayed? Such questions and their answers are completely individual, of course, but without some experience referable to them you would not be where you are.

Much of what is wondrous in medicine is communal. We are grateful for the presence of others who share our difficult journey. Even in this supportive environment, though, in matters of patient care the physician decides and acts alone—and lives alone with the results of those decisions. It is this aspect of medicine that delineates reputation from character. Reputation comes from things we do that others know about. Character emanates mostly from actions taken when no one else is looking. My experience convinces me that the great majority of physicians value character far above reputation. They also know the cost of possessing it, a cost not even those closest to us can truly comprehend. Understanding the solitary price paid, perhaps what a physician should be most grateful for is the individual self—for being what physicians are: intrepid, faithful, compassionate, uncompromising in matters of patient care.

If you can be totally candid for a moment and contemplate the following quote without pretense or false humility, you may recognize someone you know. Written to describe the face of *The Dying Gaul*, it could as well have been written about healers throughout time, and no less in ours:

*What we can rely on are the comeliness and iron virtue of the short-lived hero: his loyalty to cause and comrades, his bravery in the face of overwhelming odds, the gargantuan generosity with which he scatters his possessions and his person and with which he spills his blood.*

This likely describes you. If so, like the soldiers on the pool deck you have paid a great price to do a great good and have helped more than you can know. Please accept my admiration and gratitude. Knowing that you are along on the journey feels like the warmth of the sun.[1]

––––––––

*The Dying Gaul* is an ancient Roman marble copy of a lost Hellenic Sculpture, which was probably done in bronze in 230–220 BCE. The marble statue depicts a wounded Celtic warrior with a bleeding sword puncture visible in his lower right chest. He lies, leaning on one arm, on his fallen shield with his sword lying beside him, signifying that he knows he will die. The statue serves both as a reminder of defeat, and as a memorial to his bravery. *The Dying Gaul* is placed in the Capitoline Museum in Rome.

––––––––

[1] Hergott L. Galileo's Grapes: Recognizing Those Who Helped Make Us Who We Are. *JAMA*. 2003;290:2235–2236.

# Essays and Poems
# Manifesting the *Soul of Medicine*

# DEVOTION IN A TIME OF MOURNING

Forlornly aware of the mantles we bear
in various states of duress,
my heart warmly bounds
as I see all around
our silent pronouncement of,
"Yes."

———————

# THE TIME OF THE THREE DYNASTIES

*From the time of the Three Dynasties men have been running
in all directions. How can they find time to be human?*

– Chuang Tzu

My brother-in-law David died last week. He was 41. No one knows
exactly how the accident occurred, but his family, and other farmers,
could guess the specifics and especially the cause. He had a wife and
six young children, worked three crop farms, kept some cattle, looked
after his mother and her place, and was the executor of his uncle's
contested will. Even to a doctor he seemed enormously overextended.

David's wife said his sleeping habits had suffered noticeably for
months because of the pressures he felt, and he slept little the night
before he died. Yet he worked all the next day, and on that midsummer
evening—feeling there was still more that had to be done—he took a
tractor mower and went to clear some thick brush around the fields of
his mother's farm. A line of fence wire got caught in the large blade and
at 8:30 p.m., knowing better, he positioned himself under the heavy
piece of equipment to free the wire. Then something shifted, slipped,
and he died. There could be no sophisticated medical intervention, not
even a resuscitation. He was dead within a few horrible minutes, his
chest crushed, his mother there to witness it after his agonized call. The
sight of his lifeless body was so disturbing that the people gathered at
the scene would not allow his wife to look at him but only to hold his
cold hand as it lay exposed at the edge of the tarp that covered him.

It took six men to lift the mower off his body.

The pain of his family was indescribable, unknowable even in its
essence except perhaps by others who have had a similar loss. There had

been no similar loss for these sufferers, though. Nothing they had experienced could assist them in their grief, nothing could assure them that the pain they felt was survivable. In the early days after David's death, his wife's face reflected more daze than anguish; his children were more fidgety than tearful, at least in their public moments. Those of us around them knew that we could fill their time but that there was really nothing substantial we could do to fill the void his death had caused. Some in his community, perhaps not knowing what else to say, remarked, "Life goes on." Yes, but never in the same way for those who loved him most.

Was David overworked? Under too much stress? Finally careless? Almost surely "yes" to all of these. Everyone who knew him wondered whether he had to die. Were there not at least a few critical periods when he could have stepped back, seen differently, changed his course, and perhaps saved his life?

For physicians, is there a lesson here? The similarities, you must agree, are striking: heavy, often isolated, and (seemingly) imposed workloads; the pressures of time, achievement, income, and other responsibilities; the primacy of work over all other interests, although the principals often claim otherwise. This was David's reality, and it is also ours. What drives us to it? As humans in the early 21st century, our identity seems largely defined by what we have, what we do, and how we learned to do it. We understand ourselves this way, too. Physicians may be examples of the very worst kind, typically taking not only our work—and ourselves—too seriously but also working too long, too intensely, and at a pace we would never advise or even allow our patients to maintain. In medicine, at least, there is a point beyond which this behavior is hypocrisy, not valor. How much work and reward are enough? How much is too much? Who has control? Do we know the real cost? Who pays the price?

When I was a medical resident, I began to hear bothersome comments from older physicians about the practice of medicine after the training years. "Medicine is a jealous mistress," one professor commented, reflecting, among other things, the male dominated medical structure of the time. "I always tell the residents' wives not to expect that the long hours, absence from the home, and hard work will change once their husbands go into practice," he said. This was the same man whose wife had found an undelivered letter in their daughter's bedroom drawer after she went away to college, telling him that over the years he had sacrificed his family for the sake of his medical practice and had thus stolen something from her. (Another letter, forgiving him years later, was carried daily in his briefcase for the rest of the time I knew him.)

Other quotes about medical practice stayed in my memory and communicated recurring, dissonant themes. A partner in a hectic cardiology practice I joined made the following statement—memorable especially for its prophetic latter phrase—to my wife when a sprinkler head on our lawn didn't work: "Well, you had better learn to take care of these things yourself, because he's not going to be here."

Also telling is a quote from my wife to a neighbor when I left that practice and came to Denver by myself for a month to find a house for our family: "What's it like to have my husband gone? Well, it's not much different from when he was here."

A prominent cardiovascular surgeon in Houston, the editor of at least one surgical text, told me that his goal when he left the house each morning was to get back before the 10:00 p.m. news. "I never made it," he said, and after several years of this he finally gave up a very lucrative and prestigious practice in cardiovascular surgery for one in preventive medicine. I last saw him here in Denver a few years ago with his wife, watching their son play college lacrosse. I think of him as one of the most courageous physicians I have ever met. His willingness to undergo not only a change in type of practice but also a deeper, more radical change in personal and professional identity is admirable.

Other stories over the years—usually told in a matter of fact, lamentable tone or with outright nostalgia during placid moments in the doctors' lounge—reinforced these early impressions. A senior cardiologist's daughter told him, "We don't remember you until we were about 8 years old, because that's when we were old enough to stay up until you got home." Another doctor invited a grown daughter to spend an afternoon with him and was told, "You know, Dad, you didn't have time for me when I was young, and now I don't have time for you."

Finally, when one of my cardiology partners was in an earlier, busier practice and was gone much of the time, his son asked his mother, "Did Daddy die?"

My Midwest medical school's 20-year reunion information form requested data not only on the location and type of practice the graduates had but also information about their spouses:

#1. _____

#2. _____

These vignettes are all about accomplished and upright individuals who are of great service to their patients. The stories' theme of imbalance and its consequences does raise the question, however, about whether our professional focus is one of the "shadows cloaked in light" that Baltasar Gracian warned us about in the 17th century. Are we so dedicated to the unquestionably honorable mission of enhancing the lives of our patients that in some ways we actually impede—or harm— the lives of others, including ourselves?

At my brother-in-law's wake, several people commented that life is short. Short or not, as a Tibetan Buddhist friend pointed out, life is finite, each moment irretrievable, and although we know this we don't believe it. If we did, our behavior would change. We wouldn't waste time in any way, especially in overwork and preoccupation and stress. Almost anyone who has had a serious threat to his or her life or health will confirm this. As my brother-in-law's death shows, these things are killing our sensibilities, our culture, and ourselves.

David's neighbors would say that besides being a hard worker, he was also lucky, inheriting good land, farm machinery, buildings, and money. Like us, he got his wish, but somehow it all became too much to handle. With him it might have been the result of expectations based on the work habits of generations of farmers before him, coupled with his own way of coping. He had imagined no other way. Eventually it all became harmful—fatally for him and horribly for his family.

I think it's so with many physicians, too, who would otherwise not identify with him. Amidst all the excitement, professional satisfaction, glory, and possessions, there is often an awareness of some profound yet distressing reality that these things cannot satisfy: perhaps an illness; an awareness of children "suddenly" grown and distant; spouses often gone or at least living separate lives; some of us, perhaps finally introspective, longing for opportunities missed. Golden handcuffs are still handcuffs. Our "successes" call to mind a passage in the Tao Te Ching that speaks of a water-bearing vessel that tips over when filled to the brim but remains upright when filled to a lower level.

All is not darkness in the practice of medicine, certainly. Besides its inherent value to our patients, the very privilege of participating in it, the sense of achievement felt after completing seemingly countless years of study and sacrifice, the satisfaction and humility generated by assisting others in a time of need, and the opportunity to provide well for one's loved ones are just a few of the benefits that come to those in its service. Not surprisingly, many argue that there is not a widespread problem with the way the modern medical life is lived, or, considering the degree and pace of change in its practice, that there is little we can do to gain control over it. Others insist that there is still much we have to learn about how to do it well.

Is there imbalance in our individual practice of medicine? Do we need to "save ourselves from the world of our time," as Thomas Merton suggested? Are the principles and ideals required for balance irreconcilable with millennial realities? We each have to answer this for ourselves, taking the time to think about it at all, of course. For me, lessons learned over the years from my own and others' experiences have evoked a profound understanding of and appreciation for what I value at the deepest level, as well as philosophical and practical changes based on that awareness: continuing the commitment to excellence in patient care yet valuing relationships with loved ones over professional concerns; taking Wednesdays off; dissociating myself from a consuming practice; ceasing to do interventional cardiology; getting involved in community work; and committing to a simpler lifestyle. The effect of making these sometimes-difficult choices has been a less remunerative but otherwise richer and more vivid life for my family and myself.

But in this plurality there is no simple or uniform answer to why we structure our days or ourselves the way we do. A specific occurrence like my brother-in-law's tragic death compels some level of personal reflection for all of us who knew him and, however horrible, can have meaning for others as well. His life and death speak strongly to me, and I hear more as time passes: life is finite; we are driven, often by things inapparent; we cope—sometimes not in the best way, although we may think in the only way; our actions not only affect but define others; and, even with the enormous amount of information and experience in our consciousness, we are all too often shamefully unaware of happenings in even our most intimate relationships, let alone elsewhere. In epidemiologic terms, the condition of imbalance in the practice of medicine seems to me pervasive enough to be considered endemic and even stereotypic. Its recognition and treatment, of course, are intensely personal.

How are you? And yours? What would they say? Do you dare ask them?[2]

--------

[2] Hergott L. The Time of the Three Dynasties: Reflections on Imbalance in the Practice of Medicine. *Annals of Internal Medicine.* 1998;128:149–151.

# LOST IN A DARK WOOD

*It is difficult to get the news from poems*
*Yet men die miserably every day for lack of what is found there.*

– William Carlos Williams, "Asphodel, That Greeny Flower"

Difficult in any era, the practice of medicine today seems accompanied by so much unhappiness I am convinced that if clinicians en masse took the Minnesota Multiphasic Personality Inventory, there would be a significant elevation of scale 2 (depression). If there were a "medicine as fun" scale, it would be inversely decreased, with the largest decrement in the scores of those who have practiced for more than a decade. This is unfortunate, considering the talent and dedication of physicians, most of whom simply want to do the very best for their patients, often at great cost to themselves and their loved ones. Applying what the poet David Whyte said of the corporate world, we too are living in medicine the opening line of Dante's Inferno: "In the middle of the road of my life I awoke in a dark wood where the true way was wholly lost" (Sayers/Reynolds translation). One of my concerns is that as physicians progressively alter their medical practices to deal with the extraneous "market" forces acting on them, they are displaced further from "the true way." Worse, we may forget where we were heading in the first place: toward fulfilling a life vow to serve those in need, a goal that too often now seems more burden than privilege. Yet, another wisdom text offers hope—and direction. The 2500-year-old Tao Te Ching reminds us that "he who does not lose his station will endure."

What is our current station? Have the core values and goals of medicine changed, even from the recent past? How do we reconnect with who we are professionally, after spending a distracting decade focused more on what we do and how we do it? Thomas Merton would have described us as "prisoners in the world of objects," objects here indicating not our possessions but the noncore "things" such as time and remuneration constraints and limitations on clinical decision making that pulled us into their vortex during the 1990s. And, from which we feel powerless to escape. It is from the lower realm of preoccupation with them that we must release ourselves to recognize medicine once again as a calling rather than a job and reestablish "the harmony between vocation and occupation" Sam Keen mentioned in his book, Fire in the Belly: On Being a Man.

Seeking clarification and guidance, I have been inspired by "wisdom sources" of many kinds. Wisdom sources are evocative, revealing, settling, and sustaining. Their lessons emanate from a place beyond ordinary cognition, which is where we must go to begin our return to the true way. (The term true way refers to the condition in which medical decisions are based on clinical information interpreted and applied by experts whose concern is for the person in their care. It excludes decisions, or time spent, emphasizing economics, profit, self-interest, or self-serving systems.) Without availing ourselves of the inspiration that wisdom sources foster, followed by recommitment and action, we will stay where we are, settling for less than what our patients, our loved ones, and we deserve. Failing to redirect ourselves, we will continue to "die miserably every day," as William Carlos Williams observed.

Different sources of inspiration abound for each person. Even after the hardest weeks dealing with the complexity of patients with cardiovascular disease, I never fail to be heartened especially by the second movement of Mozart's piano concerto No. 20 in D minor. Likewise, gazing at Claude Monet's Hoarfrost, painted after the death of his wife, with its isolated rowboat locked in ice on a gray day in a rivulet of the Seine, I have a deeper understanding of reality-imposed desolation. Yet, as the painting further instructs, desolation in the context of life to be lived, another season to come, the boat unlocked. Passages from diverse types of scripture place consuming issues within a larger framework of time and hope, closer to the essence of things, and make us more cognizant of the effort required to achieve a goal. Reading history can do the same. Stephen Ambrose's account in Citizen Soldiers of the capture of a hill outside the French town of St Lo by a small band of American soldiers during World War II evokes not only immense admiration and gratitude for their sacrifice, but puts our quandary in context—secondarily demonstrating what can be accomplished by committed people in dire circumstances.

And proximate lessons occur. While reading the first of a large number of echocardiograms I was scheduled to interpret some years ago, I found myself moving more quickly from image to image on the monitor screen than I usually would. I felt a need to slow down, but knew that the longer I took the later I would get home that night. A quote from Mother Teresa came to mind. Shortly after winning the Nobel Peace Prize, Mother Teresa was interviewed in Calcutta by a reporter who had witnessed her work there for several days and had seen the death and deprivation that surrounded her. "Do you really expect to be successful in your work?" the reporter finally asked. Mother Teresa replied, "We are not called upon to be successful. We are called upon to be faithful."

I rewound the videotape.

Isn't faithfulness a principle that should guide physicians? By the very nature of our profession, it is to our patients that we must be faithful and for the most part we are. Exceptions occur, however, as evidenced by the disturbing public comment recently of a physician who admitted to frequently lying to his patients regarding the real (monetary) reason he changes their medication. He acknowledged that in his practice, he, as a physician, is in direct personal competition with the patient for the dollars designated for health care according to his group's business arrangement. Such behavior stands in contrast to Chuang Tzu's statement, relevant to the practice of medicine at the highest level: "He would blush to be in business." Primary financial motivation is unusual in my experience, but the fact that it exists indicates how far some physicians have strayed from the path. Think about what happens to a society when its most educated and humanistic individuals function as frenetic technicians in creativity killing systems. Think about what a culture loses when people with admirable traits work so intensely on assigned tasks that little energy is left for anything except (perhaps) an insular existence focused on one's immediate family. Think too about what future generations of physicians will be like if we do not return to the true way.

I have practiced rural family medicine, military medicine, urban interventional cardiology, and academic medicine. At every step I have seen physicians working hard (often brutally so) to serve their patients and grateful for the opportunity. Far beyond the material rewards and status medical practice brings, to be allowed into people's lives, to learn and to be a part of their stories (and for them to be a part of ours), to be able, almost always, to lessen their suffering if not restore their health, and to share their suffering when you can do neither is an honor beyond description. The fact that this involves countless days and nights and months and years and decades of arduous effort may, to others, make such a thing seem earned. But no amount of effort brings entitlement to such richness. Medical practice is a form of grace, and to diminish it is to desecrate it. Aristotle said, "The true nature of anything is the highest it can become." The true nature of the physician is not what we are living today, nor where we are heading. Whether or not our troubles were brought on by earlier inattention to society's socioeconomic needs, we have allowed our evolution and destiny to be limited. Unless we move away from what we have become, we will not only drift further from the true way but course downward in a "race to the bottom."

Wisdom sources serve to illuminate a higher path. Once there we, wiser and perhaps slightly changed, will be essentially the same as other healers throughout time. Instead of a sense of discouragement, self-preservation, and depletion that now prevails, we may then feel about medicine the way the subject in Antonio Machado's poem felt about his life:

> Last night, as I was sleeping,
> I dreamt—marvelous illusion!—
> that there was a fiery sun here in my heart.
> It was fiery because it gave warmth
> as if from a hearth
> and it was sun because it gave light
> and brought tears to my eyes.[3]

--------

[3] Hergott L. Lost in a Dark Wood: How Wisdom Sources Can Light the Way. *JAMA*. 2001;285:1938–1939.

# A SINGLE CLOUD ECLIPSES THE SUN

*"The sound of a coffin hitting earth is a sound utterly serious."*

– Antonio Machado, *The Burial of a Friend*

I think about him several times a year even now, more than 30 years later. When I do it is with uncomfortable clarity and a surge of briefly incapacitating sadness and guilt. He had come to the office at the age of 62, troubled by chest tightness and shortness of breath with exertion. Intelligent and gentle, he was the kind of person you would look forward to seeing over the years. His physical examination revealed a heart murmur suggestive of severe aortic valve stenosis (narrowing), which implied a potential reduction of blood flow to the entire body with physical effort. My training, completed just months before, had taught me that it was too dangerous to exercise such patients to assess whether or not their symptoms were cardiac in origin. Rather, cardiac catheterization to determine the severity of the stenosis and coronary angiography in preparation for aortic valve replacement were appropriate. In the practice world, though, many physicians exercised such patients routinely, and after conferring with colleagues who were my senior I put my patient on the treadmill.

Not long into the test, he suddenly said he felt very bad. He lost the rhythm of his gait and was unable to keep up with the treadmill, which we quickly stopped. Woozy and barely able to step off the belt, he turned his head up and slumped to the floor. The electrocardiogram showed a regular heart rhythm and was without evidence of a heart attack. His blood pressure was unobtainable. The pathophysiology of what had happened was obvious: exercise-induced dilation of his arteries and thus marked reduction of blood pressure in the setting of what truly was severe aortic stenosis. Also clear was the necessity of rapid resuscitation if we were to save his life. But the resuscitation was unsuccessful and he died there on the floor without regaining consciousness. Stunned, the nurses and I knelt silent and immobile next to him. But the horror was not over. I still had to phone his wife, who waited at home. Making the call was in its way as hard as witnessing his death. She too seemed a lovely person and though dazed was remarkably understanding. She related that just before he left the house he had told her, "If they put me on the treadmill I don't think I will make it." He had not expressed that to me, deferring to the judgment of his cardiologist.

I have wondered over the years how long he might have lived had we been able to replace his aortic valve successfully. Would he have been alive when I thought about him in 1990? In 2000? In 2010? Is she alive? Did she live the rest of her life alone? There are two ways the death of a loved one affects people: the dying process is one, the loved one's absence the other—and often worse. She suffered the shock of the first and the loneliness of the latter. So much in life depends on who comes beside. Their journey together ended with his coming to see me. I expressed my sorrow to her then and would again if given the chance. It is painful to write about and utterly serious still.

On occasion I envision myself kneeling at my aortic stenosis patient's side after the unsuccessful resuscitation, and hearing again the sound of his wife's voice on the phone. Doing so brings a sudden inner darkness, making real in a physical way something Balthasar Gracian described in the 17th century, *a single cloud that eclipses the sun.* But, inspired by the soul of medicine, dedicated to medical practice, and motivated by the awareness of how much good there is yet to be done, I am heartened as my workday continues and I help people, as others help me—and feel once more the warmth of the sun and the mostly brilliant blue sky that medical practice is by its nature.

# FACING OUR MISTAKES

I can think of fewer than a handful of clinical decisions made over a 40-year career that I would change if I could. Putting my aortic stenosis patient on the treadmill is one. A dire patient outcome rarely signifies negligence or misjudgment on the part of the physician. Most bad outcomes occur in the setting of totally appropriate acts by the doctor, the outcome being determined rather by factors in the patient's disease process or the innate risks of treatments. But, as with the man I put on the treadmill, there are occasions when one judgment over another can harm.

No matter the specifics of the damage done, thoughtful physicians take any harm to a patient both seriously and personally—and most seriously and personally when they feel they may have committed an error. Not to do so would be a sign of dysfunction. Guilt, self-blame, horror, sorrow, self-questioning and many other emotions are appropriate in such situations, as is the necessity of the physician to be dominated by subjectivity in clinical decision making for a time. This subjectivity carries over at least to the doctor's next many patients, and sometimes forever.

Coronary angioplasty pioneer Dr. Andreas Gruentzig told us that if we were going to do that procedure, we should "expect complications." His warning can be expanded to the practice of medicine in general: *If you are going to be a physician, deciding hourly about things that affect the health and lives of patients and their loved ones, expect some bad outcomes. They will occur, no matter how careful or how good you are.*

Recalling this is somewhat comforting when an undesirable event occurs, but we are still likely to be hard on ourselves on such occasions. Training and practice emphasize the dominant principle of *primum non nocere* (first do no harm) over all other considerations.

Board certification, recertification, or the awareness of personal clinical excellence do not change this order, though they do make us more confident and less anxious about decision making after a considerable time early in our careers. We are constantly on alert while with patients, and often in their absence if we sense that something is unfinished. Compulsion, concern, and some degree of self-questioning are hard on the physician but good for the patient. I want my physician to function this way. I recall hundreds of hours spent fretting over decisions made or to be made in complex cases. Included is the occasional return to the hospital on what began as the evening drive home, to check on one last thing; or awakening at 3 a.m., preoccupied and unable to get back to sleep if something is particularly unsettled about a patient.

Physicians have been known to leave medicine after severely injuring or causing the death of a patient. Most often, though, no matter how devastated doctors feel about harm having been done, whether they are responsible or not, that feeling and the continuing awareness of the event that caused it must eventually recede to the background of the doctor's consciousness—though, as with my aortic stenosis patient, perhaps to be carried there for a very long time. Not to have them recede at an appropriate time could disrupt the orderly thought processes physicians rely on to work through patients' problems, and could thus jeopardize the wellbeing of patients who follow. It takes courage for a physician to face patients and their loved ones after a procedure or treatment goes badly; and courage as well to soon thereafter walk into the obstetric delivery suite, intensive care unit, operating room, or clinic treatment room to care for the next person who comes along with the same condition.

Physicians try to be perfect *every time* we interact with a patient or a patient's loved ones—dedicated to never miss an important comment in a patient's story, never to miss a diagnosis, never to order or perform wrong treatment, never to harm—faithfully doing these things all day long and on many nights, every week, every month, every year for many years.

But, physicians are not perfect—though, quite remarkably, we come close—and we must accept our imperfections when they emerge. Not to do so would be to submit oneself to a consumptive, crippling guilt that could markedly limit the physician-self, and likely the self. If physicians who have harmed are to be released from the tyranny of guilt they must soulfully contemplate their part in what happened, accept their degree of responsibility, accept their humanity, forgive themselves when able and, if they are to recommit to their service of healing, accept with unease the stance described about *The Man of Tao*, in Thomas Merton's translation of the book, *The Way of Chuang Tzu*, "Disgrace and shame do not deter him." Assuming this stance, we place the heavy burden of our mistakes or disappointments somewhere deep in our center and proceed to the next room—a patient waiting.

The ability to follow these precepts—for physicians or others who have harmed—helps convert the turbulent subjectivity that follows such occurrences to the more orderly and life-serving objectivity that leads to doing good, and to a state described by Thomas Merton after such a crisis:

*A personal crisis is relative and salutary if one can accept the conflict and restore unity on a higher level, incorporating the opposed elements in a higher unity. One thus becomes a more complete, a more developed person, capable of wider understanding, empathy, and love for others, etc.*

# THE CLEARING

It came to him
just after his hand left the cold metal rail
and he began to drop.

Before,
a leaden shroud
of sadness
and separation
led him to deem
his agony no longer bearable.

So,
to end his torment,
he jumped off the Golden Gate Bridge.

What came to him as he fell,
tumbling and flailing,
was a thought unexpected—
"The only real problem in your life
is that you just jumped off the Golden Gate Bridge."
He saw the thing that mattered,
that made the rest disperse,
that needed attention utterly.

Having seen,
he fought to right himself,
did,
and lived.

Seeing the thing that mattered—
and righting himself—
he lived.[4]

––––––

[4]Hergott L. The Clearing. *Ad Libitum, Annals of Internal Medicine.* 2017; 166(10):732.

# PLAYING THE MOONLIGHT
# SONATA FROM MEMORY

*Celebrating the Wonders of Our Difficult Life*
*Give wine. Give bread.... Sit. Feast on your life.*

– Derek Walcott, "Love After Love"

There is a peculiar dissociation between the intense awareness doctors have while addressing clinical problems and our barely noticing when things go well. Except for marking the clinical result as an end point, physicians seem to have selective neglect when good things occur, or at least an inability to dwell on them. Taking satisfaction in what works is not the way we operate. Most physicians would have to force themselves to think in any detail about excellent outcomes—including suffering, disability, and premature death spared by the correct application of clinical data—that they experience regularly. We remember forever the suture that tore through, the obstetric delivery that went bad, or advancing the angiographic catheter 1 millimeter too far. But we quickly forget the decision to order a lung scan that clarifies the diagnosis and saves a life in a subtle case of pulmonary embolism. Or proceeding with a biopsy on a doubtful skin lesion that turns out to be melanoma. Or the decision most often successfully made, not to test at all but to depend on our clinical assessment, itself based on expertise we also take for granted but which is in fact the product of intensive, prolonged, and ongoing study and practice. Perhaps it is because we expect to succeed almost every time that we barely notice when we do. It is the preponderance of our successes over any failures, after all, that allows us to continue in the difficult life of medical practice.

Our enjoyment of that life is rapidly decreasing. When we got our wish and set out in medicine, we assumed that it would be essentially what it had been—perhaps even better. For more than a decade, though, we have been in uncharted territory, living out what the inscription on medieval maps said of such places: "Here do be monsters." We have been pressured to respond to the very real monsters of time and remuneration constraints, and limitations on clinical decision making, by focusing dominantly on the scientific and biomedical aspects of patient concerns rather than also addressing subjective matters patients have. Doing so, we at times function more as technicians than physicians, unhappy in the bargain.

Progressively more insular and concerned about the effect the workday has on us, we are too often heedless of part of medicine's essence: celebrating with patients and their families, colleagues and staff, and our loved ones the wonders beyond the biomedical that medicine brings. We should be feeling what mythologist Joseph Campbell described as a consequence of the hero's journey: "From sacrifice, bliss." Most physicians would be hard put to claim that state of being currently, but its lack is an aberration, working toward its return a necessity.

A statement I made at the end of a British Broadcasting Corporation (BBC) video, *Healing the Hearts of Men and Gorillas*—dealing with a team of clinicians from the University of Colorado School of Medicine treating animals at the Denver Zoo is similar to Joseph Campbell's statement: "The trouble we are having in the United States, doctors, is that we are often practicing medicine as *prose* rather than the *poetry* it really is."

The wonders of medicine are ubiquitous but, like the instant in time the Impressionists captured, fleeting and easily missed if one is preoccupied. Some of my most powerful memories are images of medical personnel extending themselves to help patients and each other: a nurse standing at the bedside holding a patient's hand upon his awakening the morning after coronary artery bypass graft surgery; another nurse, kneeling on the floor with the head of a patient who had passed out while walking around the ward resting on her lap as she soothed him; my walking into the echocardiography reading room in the evening and coming upon partners, themselves intensely busy, who had stayed late to help interpret echoes that were my responsibility but which I couldn't get to until then.

A patient with severe dilated cardiomyopathy once told me after his being started on a dobutamine drip, "You've given me back my sense of humor." He did not mention the increased energy he had, nor his newfound ability to sleep through the night without awakening short of breath. The treatment result with the most meaning for him was beyond the purely physiologic. His sense of humor's return was a cause for celebration in his view.

In the last week of my 10 years of medical training a 75-year-old man came to cardiology clinic who had a prosthetic aortic valve implanted in his heart 12 years before. The patient felt good physically and emotionally. He was pleased that he felt so good after such a long time with a prosthetic valve, and wondered if there were any valvular abnormalities after that long a time.

On examination his prosthetic valve sounded fine and, to his great relief, I was pleased to tell him there was no valve dysfunction, and that he could do anything he wanted to physically. I asked him to come back to the clinic in a year to have his valve checked again.

After he left the clinic I wondered how often the artificial leaflets of that valve had opened and closed over those years. At his heart rate of 72 beats per minute, I was stunned to discover that every 24 hours the valve had opened and closed 103,680 times. At that pulse rate, every 10 days the heart would have beaten over one million times, every month over three million times, and every year over 36 million times. I was astounded that, for the duration of its service to him, the valve— functioning normally still, demonstrating the success of treatments and the faithfulness of the beating heart—had opened and closed *over 447 million times*!

One physician-patient, an accomplished pianist, silently worried after suffering an acute myocardial infarction and undergoing emergency coronary bypass graft surgery in the middle of the night, whether he would still be able to play Beethoven's *Moonlight Sonata* from memory. The first seat he took when he got home was in front of his grand piano, where he played it through "by heart." Such stories are cherished by those who live them. No matter what the pressures of the day, we should not exclude ourselves from experiencing and celebrating them. Indeed, without such experiences why would anyone begin or stay on our path?

Having had a long career as an invasive cardiologist prior to joining the faculty of a medical school, I am often asked by residents and fellows about the practice world. I tell them that when they go into practice they should expect to work very hard all of the time, and brutally hard some of the time. I advise them to avoid any practice that expects them to work brutally hard a lot of the time. Such a practice triggers "survival" behavior contrary to the well-being of the physician, his or her loved ones, the greater community, and, ultimately, patients. Such a practice dictates that medicine be lived as prose rather than the poetry it is by nature.

I also tell them that there will be periods of self-doubt and remorse, that some memories will haunt them, but that the benefits to self and especially to others of such a life make it well worth living. My hope for them is that they experience and treasure for a very long time the best of what it is to *be* a physician.

A Hopi image depicts a person standing at the end of a maze that symbolizes the course of a life, looking back and seeing that it was, after all, good. At the end of our careers hopefully we will feel the same. Waiting until then to observe and introspect, though, means missing a lot along the way. Perhaps it is best, amidst the twists and turns, the hills to climb with loads to carry, feeling tired and lost, to at times take Derek Walcott's advice. Pause. Look around. Contemplate what we are really about. And feast on the goodness of such a life.[5]

--------

[5] Hergott L. Playing the Moonlight Sonata From Memory: Celebrating the Wonders of Our Difficult Life. *JAMA*. 2002;288:2516–2517.

# THE DESKTOP PHOTO

The small photograph that sits alone on the office desk of a surgical colleague tells a life-saving story. Indicative of its importance to him, the photo has rested on his desk since the day he first occupied the office nearly a decade ago. Like the other artifacts he has placed around the room, though, each chosen for its meaning or its beauty, over time the photo has assumed a background role. He hardly notices the objects as he does his work there. Attention is directed instead toward papers that cross his desk, images that come and go on his computer screen, work on the phone, staff and colleagues entering and leaving, and ever-present thoughts in between about clinical or administrative issues. But the manner in which he attends to these tasks, the way he treats his patients, even how he performs their operations, has much to do with the stories the artifacts tell. They are reflective of the formative and sustaining things he has experienced that make him the doctor and person he is. On a recent occasion he did take the picture off his desk to look at it, and what it conjured up brought him to tears. For the life saved in the story the picture tells is not the life of a patient, but of his own family.

The picture shows two little girls in their pajamas sitting on a bed holding a telephone. They are saying good night to him, their father, still at work. This they commonly did since he was a member of a group that scheduled operations well into the evening. Present in the scene, though not in the picture, is the girls' mother, who took the photo for reasons and feelings of her own. The scene speaks of innocence, separation, unfortunate and recurring compromise—and hints at possible regrettable future realities.

Inscribed on the picture are the words 'Thank You Daddy'—an obscure inclusion, until he explains 'Thank You Daddy' was written by the girls later, the picture then framed and presented to their father in thanks for his leaving that practice for one that allowed him to be home most evenings. The completed scene speaks of caring, responsiveness, optimism and wholeness.

The photo serves as an emotive reminder for him of what was and might have been—and of what is, the family together and well, and he perhaps the most thankful of all for having made the decision he did.[6]

———

[6] Hergott L. Desktop Photos. *Canadian Medical Association Journal.* 2006; 175:781.

# THE VIEW FROM FIESOLE

*Close both eyes*
*to see with the other eye.*

– Jelaluddin Rumi

Some of the younger members of a large cardiology group are pressing to shorten the time allotted to see office patients, claiming, "The more patients we see, the more money we make." They want 15 minutes for a return visit and 30 minutes for a new patient consultation.

A cardiologist from another city called to see if our university group was hiring. When I asked why he was interested in joining us, he said, "You know, to make it in the private world these days you have to sell your soul. And I'm not sure I want to do that."

At a recent party, when I asked an interventional cardiologist friend with adolescent children how his practice was going, and particularly whether his workload was too heavy, he said after a reflective pause, "It's just about right." Visiting with his wife later in the evening, I asked her the same question. She responded, "Well, like tonight, I always appreciate it when people invite our children too. It's really catch-up time for the kids and their dad."

On the first day of Orientation Week for first-year medical students, our dean asked the students how many of them had been advised by at least one physician not to go into medicine. Eighty percent of the students raised a hand.

I have been increasingly concerned about the effects of external forces imposed on physicians in the last decade. My concern includes not only the obviously diminished autonomy of physicians, but also what seems to be lessened organizational and cultural value of physicians. More bothersome are some of the responses physicians have made to the pressures.

Understanding the interests of the parties imposing these forces—interests largely driven by economics and profit—and understanding that physicians have historically not been sufficiently attentive to the financial implications of health care delivery, this devolution of medicine must be reversed, not just for us, but for the welfare of patients, our loved ones, future physicians and our culture. A fundamental step in reversing our insidious diminishment is to recognize that there is something more than physician autonomy and valuation at risk. Some of the imposed pressures, and some of the responses to them, threaten to extinguish the soul of medicine—that thing beyond the biomedical, immutable, sustaining: the caring, compassionate, dedicated, enthusiastic attitude that set us on the difficult-by-nature, enriching journey called the medical life. Engrossed as so many of us are in our workday activities, perhaps we need to consider a profoundly different way of seeing if we are to preserve the soul of medicine—seeing with our "other eye," as Rumi declared, the eye of the soul. I offer as a means for us to see differently the metaphor of the view from Fiesole.

I have learned that most people are not familiar with Fiesole, or what can be experienced there. Fiesole is in Tuscany, just a few miles up a hill from Florence. Galileo and many other notables spent time there, including John Milton, who mentioned Fiesole in Paradise Lost. Either because of lack of knowledge of the town, or not wanting to bother to leave Florence and go there, comparatively few travelers visit Fiesole. For those who make the effort, wonders await—especially the enchanting, almost unbearably picturesque scene of Florence resting silent and majestic in the valley below. In her New York Times review of Francine Prose's The Lives of the Muses, the author Stacy Schiff listed some things in the current era she felt serve as muses—as in ancient Greece, entities that inspire creativity in the arts and humanities. One thing listed was love. Another was suffering. A third was the view from Fiesole.

Why Florence and Fiesole in a discussion of the preservation of the soul of medicine? I am going to ask that we consider being in Florence a metaphor for our day-to-day experiences in medicine, and the view from Fiesole a metaphor for stepping out of that awareness, at least in our minds, and perceiving those experiences in a broader, more soulful way—a view beyond biological science; a view that emphasizes our relationships to our patients, our loved ones, and ourselves.

I do not offer the metaphor of taking the view from Fiesole as something merely interesting. I offer it, or something like it, as being essential—to the preservation of the soul of medicine, and thereby to the enhancement of the lives of physicians. I offer stepping away and taking a more soulful perspective as a career saver, a lifesaver, a way to escape, not just for the moment but long term, the rush, entrapment, and depletion many physicians feel much of the time. I do not offer being in Florence bad, and taking the view from Fiesole good. I offer both as what they are, fundamental and sustaining, neither being sufficient but both being necessary.

Being in Florence would be finishing work and heading home, spent from the efforts of the day. The returning home ritual might begin with the closing of the car door, and a sense of relief at finally being alone, and continue with barely noticing the same sights on the same drive taken innumerable times before, perhaps accompanied by the routine distraction of music or news on the radio. The ritual might end with the turn onto the driveway to the house, and the greeting of loved ones.

Taking the view from Fiesole would be to occasionally ponder and always understand that beyond our more obvious day to day struggles, separate battles are being fought by those we love, benevolently engaged in them because of their devotion to us. As well as providing much in the way of benefit, medicine by its nature and throughout its course calls on all of its participants to sacrifice in the name of others. A physician's spouse or soulmate, and children, live that reality deeply. They are the ones kept waiting time and time again as the physician's estimate of arrival time home from work, intended to be precise, is understood by them as a loose approximation, with the arrival and the start of whatever activity they are planning likely to be delayed even further. Medical families know too the disappointment of treasured occasions being diminished due to the absence of one of their members;

like the chair saved at the school play remaining empty as the play progresses, and the fleeting, sigh-inspiring vision of the costumed child's expression able to be burnished only on the souls of those present. Yet perhaps during that absence, a different person's life is saved, the course of an illness reversed, or pain relieved.

The view from Fiesole includes a deep appreciation for the struggles of those we love, for the goodness of their work, and for the sense of warmth that contemplation of their presence in our lives brings.

I am not naive to the difficulty of being fully present to patients and others. I have felt the pressures that make such presence difficult and on occasion have experienced survival behavior, and lived medicine at work and at home as prose rather than the poetry it is by its nature. I have spent more time dwelling in Florence than was necessary or good.

But I have lived in medicine something far different the great majority of the time, inspired and reassured by its wonders and its goodness, the "other eye" aware in the diligence of the work. I have learned from the work and the wonders that what is life giving—to my patients, my loved ones, and myself—is not only what I do but who I am. I have seen that the preservation of the soul of medicine is also the preservation of the soul of the physician, and that both are essential if one is to feel oneself a physician. My hope is that with the attention we will pay to the preservation of both, the 80% of students who raised a hand will not advise those who follow as they were advised, and that they will feel about their lives in medicine the way the stars in another Rumi poem felt:

> The stars come up spinning
> every night, bewildered in love.
> They'd grow tired
> with that revolving, if they weren't.
> They'd say,
> "How long do we have to do this?"[7]

--------

[7] Hergott L. The View From Fiesole. *JAMA*. July 10, 2013;310(2):147–148.

# LOVING HER

I had a patient who,
for years
after his wife of many years
died,
went to her grave daily.

He didn't go there to visit her
and then get on with his day.
Visiting her was his day,
and he spent it sitting in a chair
near her,
or what was left of her,
in the ground
and in his heart.

He must have spoken to her
throughout the day—
would that be monologue or soliloquy?
I'm sure to him it was a conversation.

Why did he do it?
I never asked,
perhaps assuming I understood.

Whatever his reasons,
he described his days contentedly.

Clinical concerns aside,
loving you as I do,
I was happy for him.[8]

———————

[8] Hergott L. Loving Her. *Ad Libitum, Annals of Internal Medicine.* 2015;163:51.

# COURAGE AND THE JOURNEY
# THROUGH THE FOREST

Courageous acts are typically thought of as being dramatic, vividly recalled, and of relatively brief duration even when they are life changing. While such a characterization often fits the remarkable courage shown by patients and their loved ones when they are suddenly called upon to deal with a health catastrophe, it less often describes the times when doctors manifest courage. Courageous acts by physicians emanate from traits like compassion, duty, and commitment, qualities that doctors apply daily throughout their careers and exhibit long before they lay hands on a patient. Each of us can recall, for example, the undergraduate pursuit of medicine calling for submission to a vast academic regimen that sacrificed other scholarly interests and social opportunities, with the risk that after years of intense collegiate or even postgraduate focus admission to a medical school may be denied. All of these and more are considered for a plainly honorable but otherwise vaguely understood existence at the end of the quest. For an individual pondering whether to venture forth, it is at the point of sensing how daunting and uncertain the journey can be that courage is first called for. Reflective of this, I find great meaning in something I read about what the Old French text of *The Quest of the Holy Grail* describes when, if a knight wants to succeed, he must enter the forest "at a point that he, himself, had chosen, and where it was darkest." At some point long before, every physician of today summoned the amount of courage necessary and stepped into the forest.

As experienced physicians will affirm, those who have been successful in the first part of their quest enter medical school and find that the journey becomes unimaginably more difficult—initially because of

the colossal amount of information students are required to assimi-
late in the first two years, and later as they assume the responsibilities
of clinical decision making. Especially early in their medical education these realities are again experienced as dark and disorienting
by many. A student graduating with honors from our medical school
related recently that, "If you're not in a total state of shock your first
few months of medical school you don't understand what's going on."
Yet, medical students persevere, making frequent use of what may be
called *buttocks power* (the discipline of sitting for extended periods of
time over texts and other resources that slowly divulge their exotic con-
tents). As medical students and later in their training they tolerate the
inadequacies and sometimes-archaic traditions of medical education,
including the diverse, not always pleasant or helpful, and occasionally
harmful, personalities of people to whom they are academically subser-
vient. They may stumble or become distracted but refuse to be moved
from the laudable course to which they are committed. Throughout,
the trainees continue to forfeit much along the way, heeding the attes-
tation of their professors that a great deal is asked of them because the
stakes are so high for people who will be in their care. As is generally
true of physicians at any stage, the trainees' loads are lightened, and
the forest brightened, by the companionship and support of colleagues
moving toward the same destination and operating from the same set of
ethereal principles. True as well of more experienced physicians, those
in training are sustained by the continual unfolding of the wonders of
medicine and their application to the wellbeing of others. Yet, the path
is often solitary, rarely level, and at times courses through literal and
metaphorical darkness and cold. What may not even be recognized as
courage nonetheless continues to be called for.

At the beginning of the journey, hopeful individuals step into the
forest declaring an ardent desire to be a doctor. Since many at that
point have little practical understanding of what a doctor's life is like
I think what the hopefuls actually mean is that they want to *become* a
doctor. They want to get into medical school and get their degree. They
will then go on to live the medical life, whatever that turns out to be for
them. As arduous as the becoming phase is, the decades-long period
of *being* a physician is a deeper and broader reality understood only in

the doing, and calling for a deeper and broader kind of fortitude. Life gets more complex, with attention required to an assortment of potential issues not previously operative, or at least not to such a degree: balancing family or other personal time with that of medical practice; a change in identity from newly trained to established physician, with its attendant implications for management of finances, possible changes in self-image or even values; the breakup of a family; bearing a great sorrow or a great secret; illness; aging; etc. In the face of these and other realities doctors summon the mental, moral, and very often physical strength required to persevere, dedicated at their core to the well-being of their patients and real-life examples of Robert Frost's declaration that, "Such as we were, we gave ourselves outright."

Some practical illustrations may be clarifying. It takes courage for a physician, tired and sodden at the end of the day, to make that last patient phone call, which perhaps could have waited until morning, or to stop in at the hospital to check on a patient one final time. It takes courage on the part of physicians and their loved ones to take less financial remuneration in exchange for more time to be together. It takes unimaginable courage to continue on the path, sad and lonely, when a spouse or other treasured loved one departs. It takes a particular kind of courage, too, for a physician to recognize when a career's journey ends and walk away, down a less familiar and perhaps less enriching path, knowing that, although the hard-earned title *Doctor* remains, personal identity changes in the absence of patients to care for.

Perhaps it is when healers themselves need healing that the greatest amount of courage from them is called for; the time when the nonspecific symptom turns out to signify the one condition in the differential diagnosis we hoped it would not. It must seem eerie when physicians acquire a condition they have treated themselves, seen through a microscope, or even in a jar in the pathology laboratory. When things get serious, it must be disorienting, too, recalling the manner in which thousands of clinical decisions were made and recommendations offered to others over a career, to find oneself in the receiving role in that process.

As is commonly experienced, since about the age of forty I have noticed a crescendo in the incidence of various maladies in friends and family, and as time passes a greater frequency of their being tragic, life-ending diagnoses. Being of an age that places me in Act III of the play, *"Life"*, I wonder about whether or when current or future ailments will denote that I am in Scene 3 rather than early in Scene 1, as that untrustworthy variable *chronology* now indicates. I hope, for myself and other doctors, that when the telling symptom appears we will be rational enough to take a predominantly responsive rather than overly analytical role, wise enough to seek attention, and humble enough to put our trust in the person caring for us. As for courage in that instance, it is too uncertain to speculate about, too private to share, and will depend once again on what transpires in the cold and the dark. If physicians are fortunate enough to be able to reflect at that point, hopefully they will find strength in the recognition that their professional life from its very beginning has been replete with acts of courage. I do know that, for me at that moment of need, I will at the very least be deeply grateful to my physician for having ventured into the forest, withstanding the difficulties medicine brought, and traveling the long, hard, journey to arrive at my side.[9]

---

[9] Hergott L. The Journey Through the Forest: Reflections On Courage In the Practice of Medicine. *The Intima.* Non-Fiction—Fall 2012;1–4.

# ANGELS SMALL AND LARGE

Those of us in medicine have the gargantuan privilege of living in a reality of constant meaning, experiencing challenges and marvels in the course of our entire career that must be lived to be understood or even imagined. One of the most touching and wondrous scenes I have witnessed is perhaps the most sacred space I have entered in my career, and absolutely the saddest.

When I was on a pediatric clerkship in my third year of medical school a few other medical students and I were taken to a neighborhood residence in suburban Minneapolis. The house had been converted into a state nursing home for infants with the then-untreatable condition of hydrocephalus. The house's rooms were filled with iron cribs, in each of which lay a child with a head as big as a watermelon. The babies had to lie on their sides because they couldn't support their heads lying on their backs.

As I visited the children I bent over and tilted my head so that our faces were lined up and I could look into their eyes. Some other students and I spoke to the children in the soothing way people talk to babies around the world. The children's eyes seemed focused on me, but there was no response from them as I softly spoke—no fear, no cry, no smile, no laugh. There was just the vision of a beautiful, fixed face.

We were told that since the children came from all over the state, most of the parents who lived a long distance away no longer visited them—and that most of the parents who lived closer came less and less over time, or stopped coming entirely. The babies' time was spent, rather, in the company of angels in the form of nurses who worked in teams of two, lifting and turning each infant several times a day to avoid pressure sores on the babies' immobile and heavy heads, speaking lovingly to the children as they did so, hour after hour, day after day, night after night. It was the *presence* of the nurses, in the most profound meaning of the word, that was wondrous.

In writing about my visit with the children years later I became tearful, wondering if they were sad and lonely—as they could do nothing but lie in a crib in the company of strangers and away from their families. Still tearful, I called a wise and sensitive senior pediatrician who had cared for such children and asked him that question. He told me he couldn't be certain, but the increased pressure in the babies' skulls was so high that the cerebral cortex was markedly thinned, and that the children were thus likely neither perceptive nor cognitive. Hearing that gave me some relief.

I am also soothed that in advanced countries there are no longer such babies. Researchers devised a way long ago to lower intracranial pressure by placing small caliber tubes in the brain that drain intracranial fluid from the brain to the abdomen or the heart—a wonderful medical marvel.

Still, I sometimes sense that I am back in that house with the children, feeling the sadness of the scene but, eventually, being deeply grateful for the love the nurses imparted as they blessed us all.

--------

# BLESSING FOR A NEWBORN CHILD

For _____

Dear One,

Now, at the beginning of your wondrous life,
may you feel in the caress of your Mother's arms
the full measure of tenderness offered,
which is absolute
and endless.

May you see in your Father's eyes
his never-ending promise to be your guide,
your protector,
your friend.

May you grow strong,
righteous,
true—
to life,
to family,
to the sustaining goodness of tradition,
to others,
to the Earth—
to yourself.

May your accomplishments
be profound,
and of service to others—

their greatness known to you
but they offered in humility.

May you find in life another
whose soul completes yours,
and may your life together be rich
and joyful.

May yours be a life of inner peace
lived in a time of peace.

May your life be long,
may you live it well,
and when you, yourself,
consider it after a time,
may you deem it—
splendid.

———————

# ALVIN

*"The things of a man for which we visit him*
*were done in the dark and the cold."*

– Ralph Waldo Emerson

My late father-in-law, an intelligent and hard-working farmer, once said to me of medicine, "Well, it's mostly just visiting, isn't it?" From his experience of going to a small-town doctor when necessary it understandably appeared so. Completely unknown to him was the decades-long, arduous journey his physician had traveled to arrive at his side. The fact that even minute parts of that journey—which at times coursed through literal and metaphorical darkness and cold—remained hidden from my father-in-law as the physician demonstrated one of the characteristics that the best doctors manifest and communicate to their patients: "When we are together, there is no one and no thing in the world but the two of us." The patient is the focus of attention no matter what the physician's journey, including personal burdens he or she may carry into the examination room. Essentially, the physician is present as expert counselor and servant to the patient. It is the patient's story told and only questions about the patient's story asked in an attempt by the physician to reassure the patient that all is well if it is, restore that person's health if it is not, or share in the suffering that ensues if the news is seriously bad. In such interactions, the patient is the subject utterly. The *I* of the physician, typically robust, is subjugated to that of the patient to the point of its perceived eradication.

Not all such patient-doctor interactions are as enlightened as that. In the current context of medical practice, extraneous forces such as insurance company and hospital policies impose intense pressures on physicians that make it difficult for them to both deliver comprehensive quality care based on the physical needs of patients and attend to the social or emotional needs their conditions have brought. These limits include everything from practitioner remuneration to the time allowed to spend with a patient. One internist, who soon thereafter gave up clinical practice to go into administration, told me that with the time he was allotted to see patients he could attend to their biomedical needs but not their personal ones. I believe that most physicians chose a medical career out of a love of science and a desire to help people. The impositions that extraneous forces place on a doctor's ability to wholly realize the latter cause harm to both physician and patient. Physicians long for the return to a state of light where doctors can be concerned about the overall welfare of the one in need with whom they are face-to-face.

Until then, these and other factors can bring the doctor's needs—and thus self—into the office examination room or patient hospital room, contaminating not only the transcendent-by-nature reason the physician is there, but also changing the reality of who is the subject of their interaction. The failure to attend to a patient's needs *beyond the biomedical*—where much of the art and therapeutic potency of medicine lie—attenuates a doctor's helpfulness. It takes time and effort to communicate care and feeling to patients and others whom physicians encounter during the workday, and many doctors—perhaps understandably but still unfortunately—feel the necessity of including their needs into such interactions in order to simply get through their day. In doing so, the unidirectional flow of attention medicine calls for by its nature is diverted. Doctors in general hope for the day when that interactional flow is vigorous and praiseworthy again.

--------

# THE IMPORTANCE OF THE RIGHT HEART

The poet Wallace Stevens suggested that "Perhaps the truth depends upon a walk around the lake." Beyond the intuitive sense his statement makes, that concept has veracity for me since it was on a similar excursion, a casual drive through the countryside, that I gained an insight so evocative it eventually led to a change in how I practice medicine.

A friend who is a classical musician was explaining to the rest of us in the car a direction Beethoven had given to the players of the second movement of one of his middle string quartets, Opus 59, No. 2—a movement Beethoven reportedly found so soulful that he was brought to tears as he composed it. " '*Si tratta questo pezzo con molto di sentimento*,' Beethoven told us," our friend said. "Treat this piece with great feeling." Applications of the direction beyond its relevance for musicians came immediately to mind, including many for those of us in medicine: "Treat this patient, or family member, or student, or colleague with great feeling." What a lovely principle from which to function; but one that the difficulty of simply getting through our day may make hard to follow. Pondering Beethoven's statement further, I recalled an extraordinary clinical case about which "feeling" is one of my most vivid memories.

A small team of physicians and technicians had been asked to perform comprehensive cardiovascular examinations on the great apes at our local zoo. In captivity, nonhuman primates often die of cardiovascular conditions like those humans experience, and the examinations were part of a national program to detect and treat such conditions. All had gone well until we began our seventh session, an examination on a large adult orangutan named Penari.

Our protocol for examinations called for the animal to be anesthetized in a cage and then transported to the small zoo hospital. When Penari's sedation began to take effect, she slid to the floor in the sitting position, her back resting against the heavy iron door to the cage. The need to wait several minutes for her to become sufficiently sedated for handling and transport, as well as her position against the door, caused a delay in her medical team reaching her. During those several minutes her head had slumped forward, cutting off her airway. When she was brought to the zoo hospital, Penari was in distress with pulmonary edema and respiratory acidosis and soon became hypotensive. She was intubated and put on a ventilator, and an infusion of dopamine was begun. The diagnosis was negative-pressure pulmonary edema, its mechanism the intense negative intrathoracic pressure generated by her attempts to breathe against an obstructed airway.

Penari was treated with standard critical care modalities. Because of staffing limitations at the small hospital, her physicians took 'round-the-clock shifts at her bedside. When I arrived early one morning to start my shift I found her lead veterinarian asleep on a thin mat on the floor, his assistant standing at Penari's side. One of our cardiology fellows had slept on the mat the night before. The facility did not typically house such critically ill patients, and members of Penari's care team made several trips to community hospitals around the city securing donations of medication and equipment needed to sustain her.

Penari's oxygenation worsened, and her chest film and ventilatory dynamics suggested an early stage of acute respiratory distress syndrome. Having become quite attached to her, we were saddened that her prognosis had worsened. With further treatment, she improved to the point where an attempt at extubation was possible, but she tolerated being off the ventilator poorly. Because of the severity of her condition, its poor prognosis, and her uncertain mental status after having been in shock, it was decided that we had done all we could for her and that she would not be reintubated. She was provided comfort care, seemed not to be suffering, and died soon thereafter.

Penari was beloved by her medical team. We took her loss hard. Each of us knew that she was an innocent, a young mother who was the victim of an adverse drug reaction that killed her and left her young daughter an orphan in a social environment that may not accept her. After her death, those to whom Penari was dearest stayed the longest by her side. The cardiology fellow was inconsolable. Those caring for Penari followed Beethoven's direction well: She was treated not only with dedication and expertise but with great feeling.

The clarity of Penari's innocence made me wonder if we should consider all of our patients as such. The idea was appealing but seemed too idealistic. The answer to that question came soon thereafter when I was asked to see a patient in our hospital's burn unit. The heavily sedated young man had severe burns over most of his body, including his face. I was told that he got them when the methamphetamine laboratory he was operating exploded. Having seen the effects on others of the work of such people, a thought came immediately to my mind: "This guy got what he deserved." A glance toward the anguished look on the face of the woman standing by his side, however, made me recant and reminded me that I should have known better. I wondered what course had led her once-darling little boy to such destructive activity—and her to that heartbreaking scene. I could not categorize him as an innocent. Her look told me that he was an unfortunate, and the lesson, taken more from her look than the sight of his bandaged and weeping body, was that I should forego judgment otherwise. I gave him thoughtful and diligent care. I cannot say that it was delivered with great feeling. But, different from when I entered his room, I felt empathy for him when I left.

The contrast between my initial, reflexive judgment of this young man and the lesson his mother taught made me wonder about the wisdom of making any judgments beyond the biomedical. Judgment—positive or negative—of others seems more prevalent in our society. This appears true in medicine as well. Since physicians see more patients with "self-inflicted" diseases than we used to, for example, those who take significant amounts of medical professionals' increasingly precious time and effort to treat, some physicians may feel justified in judging or even blaming such patients for their illnesses. The epidemic of obesity is perhaps the clearest example of what some may consider a self-inflicted disease. I have seen some physicians (themselves virtually always with the body habitus of someone absent an obesity gene) express disgust at the sight or even description of some obese patients—an attitude that would be difficult to conceal from such people they treat. Alcohol abuse, smoking, illicit drug use, sexual orientation, and being indigent are other circumstances that make some patients susceptible to judgment and blame. The increasingly polarized discourse about the status of illegal immigrants is heard not only in public circles but in discussions among physicians and may put such immigrants who become patients in the same category. Judgment in perhaps its most grotesque form, fortunately as yet involving only a minority of physicians, has resulted in behaviors that most doctors consider anathema—participation in the mistreatment or torture of prisoner-patients, or even in their executions.

Some lessons are *relearned*, and the dissonance I felt recognizing my own judgments made me turn to something I dedicated myself to decades ago, but which has assumed a subliminal role in my increasingly complex life, the Oath of Maimonides. "May I never see in the patient anything but a fellow creature in pain," Maimonides wrote. The innate rightness of that statement, with its reminder of the sacred covenant being face-to-face with a fellow human in need invokes, makes judgment beyond the biomedical not only unnecessary but inappropriate.

If we are willing to take even a metaphorical walk around the lake, there are lessons to be learned, or relearned, no matter what stage of medical life we inhabit. I have concluded that not all patients are innocents. In their time of need, whether merely concerned about having a medical condition or truly affected, perhaps they may be categorized as unfortunates, and in want of what physicians are privileged to provide. I have concluded too that while possible in the great majority of cases, it is neither possible nor appropriate to treat every patient with great feeling. All patients can be treated with respect and compassion—and thus be reassured that at the very least their physician cares about their welfare. I have learned too that the separation I felt from patients I had judged was intolerable. It was this sense of separation, finally, that made me step away from the precipice and move toward a truer path—one that allowed me to fulfill a sacred vow, and to feel again the goodness of a final lesson, something Chuang Tzu taught:

When the heart is right "For" and "Against" are forgotten.

Postscript: The cardiology fellow now manages a national registry of comprehensive examinations of the great apes. The musician and his colleagues in the Takacs Quartet won a Grammy for their passionate interpretation of Beethoven's middle string quartets. The fate of the burn patient, and that of his mother, is unknown, but I hope they are well.

For D.M.H., who brought the greatest learning of all.[10]

--------

[10] Hergott L. The Importance of the Right Heart. *JAMA*. 2007;297(5):447–448.

# SALA DE ESPERANZA

The sign on the hospital wall
identifying the space
begins with a Spanish phrase—
sala de espera,
waiting room.

A more symbolic phrase
may have deeper meaning
for those awaiting news of loved ones there—
sala de esperanza,
room of hope.

Those waiting
can do little but hope—
yet hope is everything to them
in that often-desperate time
of craving favorable answers
to tormenting questions.

Is he alive?
Are baby and mother all right?
Did you get it all?
Will she be able to walk,
to talk,
to come home?

The value of those in the sala de esperanza
hoping
is not to affect
the answers to such questions.

They cannot.

The value of hoping
is the clarity
of the love of those who wait
for whom they wait.[11]

———

[11] Hergott L. Sala de Esperanza. *Annals of Internal Medicine* 2012;156:66.

# CONTEMPLATING THE LOSS OF THE LAST WWII GI

Upon my entering his room for the first time, it was the patient's large chest scar that caught my eye. As he, elderly and stout, sat partially robed on his bed, the coarse lesion on his pale skin dominated his appearance. His was a thick and disfiguring scar, obviously post-traumatic, that implied chance and urgency; yet, considering its location and his longevity, reflective of some luck in the end.

"Where did you get that?" I asked gently. "Guadalcanal," the patient flatly replied, expert at ending such discussion. After another gaze at the scar I countered, "You know, we must never forget what you guys did for us." As a withdrawn stare suddenly overtook the patient's face, a barely perceptible mist came to his eyes. Just as rapidly, a profound sense of humility came to me, aware then of being in the presence of valor.

I still have no idea why a cardiology consultation took such a turn—or where my expression of gratitude to the veteran came from. I was not a World War II devotee, had not been thinking about the GIs who fought in that war, nor the families who supported them. And, the encounter with the patient preceded recent books and movies about them by at least a year. The surprise my comment elicited in me, and the response it generated in him, did result in much further thought about the GIs. I sensed some unfinished business with them—for me personally and for our society as a whole.

Time is running out on even the last GI from World War II. Having entered the world early in the course of one century, he now quietly prepares to withdraw early from the next. Swept into his young life's perilous challenge with a body that was strong and sustaining, he now likely deals with its natural degeneration in mobility, endurance, cognition, sight—fortunate if he is not as alone now as he was in the most hazardous moments of his initial great challenge. Efforts then spent defending the liberty of the masses, he now deals with the loss of some personal freedoms that disease and degeneration bring. Who is the last GI, and what does he mean to us?

My father didn't serve in World War II. An uncle served, but he never talked about his experience to me. I remember being told once that he declined to come home when offered a brief period of rest and relaxation following his training, refusing because the thought of leaving home again was unbearable. Most of my experience with GIs has been in a less familiar, clinical setting. Having practiced cardiology for many years I have experienced thousands of GIs in this way, from very early training at VA and other teaching hospitals through the entire course of my career.

An early intuition of a deeper relationship with them came during a poignant moment at our oldest child's college graduation ceremony in 1994, when a special tribute was held in honor of the 50th reunion of the class of 1944. As these men stood—approximately half of the numbers who would normally be present, we were told—a tumultuous and heartfelt standing ovation occurred, obviously expressing far more than congratulations to alumni forebears for surviving into their eighth decade.

Then I met the patient with the chest scar. I have interviewed dozens of World War II GI patients and friends in Colorado since, with each interaction enforcing the idea that what they did long ago had an ongoing yet previously underappreciated effect on the entire course of my life. And, that I am in their debt – though that was never suggested by them.

Remarkably vivid memories and feelings remain in them from their wartime experience. Also striking is the contrast between how much that period continues to dominate their thoughts and how little it means to most of the rest of us. During a conversation following his office visit recently, one 78-year-old pulled from his wallet a bright red card with an implant of the rising sun dated Sept. 2, 1945, signifying that he was on board the USS Missouri for the signing of the official

Japanese surrender. He had carried the card on his person every day for more than half a century. "My kids don't care anything about this stuff," he said. "When I die this will be thrown away."

A Normandy veteran suffering from a recent stroke—who also fought in the Battle of the Bulge, liberated concentration camps, and made it to the Elbe River—was visited in his home in Greeley, Colorado. One of his most prized of World War II artifacts—among several dropped onto his kitchen table—was a pocket-sized copy of the New Testament with a tin front cover. Given to him in December 1941 by his wife of three weeks, he carried it in his left shirt pocket for the duration of his marches and battles, "To protect my heart from a shell," he related, literally and metaphorically.

Sentimentality does not come easily to these men. It surfaces most readily when they are reminded of comrades they served with or kindnesses done to them as a result in their time in the military. "I had seven brothers," the stroke patient said, "and the men I served with were even closer to me." One hardened veteran, who joined the Marines at the age of 19 and whose unit after three years on the islands in the South Pacific, he related, was described by Eleanor Roosevelt as "not fit for civilization," was asked if he felt appreciated over the years for his time in the service. "No," he stated quickly and emphatically. Then, tears came suddenly to his eyes as he added, "Well, once one of my three sons-in-law said on Memorial Day that he was grateful for what I had done."

As you visit with them, it is apparent that each G.I. was deeply affected by the war experience. One veteran, who could have had a deferment as a farmer but enlisted because, in his words, "This was a totally righteous war," was ordered to reregister in 1949. He did so as a conscientious objector (CO), recalling that his family and friends understood but the rural Colorado draft board didn't. "How can you be a CO when you spent three years in the army?" the board member asked. "That's why," he answered.

The evolution of my personal connection with GIs continued recently during an incidental visit to Normandy. Driving toward Omaha Beach for the first time, you are at least partially prepared for the somber feeling to be experienced there. Unexpected is the beauty of the place—surely one of the world's most spectacular cliff coasts. Walking amidst the grave markers of the American cemetery you are confronted with the painful reality of the sacrifice of very young men on this and other sacred ground. Being with the slain soldiers generates a wish to express your gratitude for their sacrifice in your name. Leaving them, there, is difficult. But you realize that they must stay, and you must go.

For me, a commitment to two things shortly followed: to express my gratitude when I could to their fellow soldiers still among us; and, to never take for granted the things for which these brave men gave their lives.

The patient with the chest scar survived. Another World War II veteran, also admitted with the small myocardial infarction about the same time, was less fortunate. An acute cardiac rupture on the third day after his heart attack—in the setting of a previous coronary bypass operation in a 79-year-old who had ordered that "no extraordinary means" be expended in his care—added up to severe mitral valve leakage, irreversible shock, and death within hours.

This 10th Mountain Division war hero's past social history included more than 9000 hours of volunteer service logged in at the Denver VA Medical Center after his time in the service, and a career as a metal finisher to support his wife and children—middle-aged and graying adults now, who poignantly wept and called loudly to him as he lay intubated, paralyzed and sedated. Having several minutes alone with him near the end I gazed at him, saddened that I had nothing substantial to offer this wonderful gentleman. Doing all I could to assure his comfort, I left, awaiting the call from the medical resident which came in the predawn informing me of the patient's death.

Looking back, and reflecting on what I have learned since, I wish I had at some time said more to him. What? I would have expressed my deep gratitude for what he did long ago enabling me to be at his side to be of service to him and others, for one thing. I have imagined what else I would like to have communicated to him, and what I would like to say to my other veteran patients:

*"When I awaken, I have a different thought each morning, not the same one I would have if my family and I were not free. Our children are healthy,*

*educated and on their way to using their natural talents. There is no one watching us. We can go where we want, do what we want within the mild constraints of a civilized society, and not only think but say what we want. Our beliefs are our own, and our right to express them, or not, is protected by the very foundation of our country. I have worked very hard for a long time to be a good doctor and have been able to live out the dream of my youth. Had you not been courageous, I could not say these things. I owe a lot to you and those who went before and beside you. I want to thank you personally for that. I will never forget what you did for my family and me, and I will never take for granted the things for which you sacrificed."*

In his book, "Kennedy," Theodore Sorenson wrote that President John Kennedy made a point of visiting military personnel regularly. This was done to ensure that the sentiments expressed in a short poem Kennedy new of, allegedly inscribed on a sentry box in Gibraltar, did not become a reality during his administration. The poem reads:

> *God and the soldier all men adore,*
> *In time of danger and no more.*
> *For when the danger is past, and all things righted,*
> *God is forgotten and the old soldier slighted.*

There are lessons for us in the poem itself and in Kennedy's example. With fewer and fewer old soldiers walking among us—*in the face of the prosperity they provided*—we should take the opportunity to thank them well before the loss of the last G.I.[12]

--------

---

[12] Hergott L. "Contemplating the Loss of the Last GI From World War II," *The Denver Post*, November 7, 1999.

# ON DUTY IN THE SURGERY WAITING ROOM

Walking in, I recognized the wood floor
and furniture in the room.
Having worked in that hospital for twenty years
I had been in the room many times
attending to patients' loved ones.

This time it was I who
waited for the doctor,
and the news.

My beloved was having a medium-risk procedure.
Though not believing the legend
that medical families
have more complications than others,
I still worried about the worst,
and took a seat in the corner.

A family entered,
led by an elderly, stately man—
Irish-looking, I thought.

He was accompanied by what appeared to be
two middle-aged daughters
and a teenage granddaughter
with numerous pierced jewelry on her face and ears.

Of the four
he seemed the most concerned.
I noticed his wedding ring.

If I were on duty, I thought,
I would approach him.
"Who is it that you're waiting for?" I would ask.
"Tell me about her."

Thankful not to be on duty,
I turned away.

His daughters frequently spoke to him
as they waited.
The granddaughter told of her new boyfriend,
with whom she was quite taken.
"Well, he seems like a fine fellow,"
the grandfather said.
He later changed seats and moved toward a daughter
who was sitting near me.
After a time he turned to me
and said in an Irish brogue,
"Who is it that you're waiting for?"
"Tell me about her."

———

# A JOURNEY BEYOND IMAGINING

Let us be merry while we may, and have joy in our minds,
For sorrow can catch us whenever it pleases.

– Sir Gawain and the Green Knight

On the grey and icy morning of January 15, 2009, feedlot workers outside the town of Wray, Colorado saw a plane descend from the low-lying clouds. The workers watched as the plane passed over them, crossed U.S. Highway 385, and then, suddenly, plunged straight down and deep into the ground. The three people on board, all professional pilots, were killed on impact. One of them was my son.

---------

"I'm surprised to see you here," one of our cardiology fellows said as he took the seat next to mine in the echocardiography reading room. His comment emanated from my return to work three weeks following the death of my son, Zachary, in a plane crash last January. After a moment's reflection I responded, "I don't know where I'm supposed to be. I don't know what I'm supposed to do. I don't know what I'm supposed to say." I did know how I felt. I felt I had been thrust into a world of familiar surroundings but with an operating principle incomprehensively different from the one I thought was real days before; a world at times I considered might be a dream but knew immediately it was not, and that there would be no startled awakening to thankful relief from its horror. I felt that a new life-clock had started ticking the moment I took the call on a hallway phone in my clinic informing me of the crash, and that everything that occurred after would be tied to that moment. I felt totally flattened—physically, psychologically, spiritually. I felt that a consuming sorrow had taken control of me, a sorrow I couldn't and surprisingly didn't want to suppress—understanding utterly why it had come. I felt out of place any time I was away from home and family, and wanted to be only there and only with them. Beneath the veneer of seeming to go through my day relatively unencumbered I felt like crying, almost all the time.

I did not weep sitting by the cardiology fellow that day, but did on scores of other occasions at work over the next months. I wept nearly any time I was by myself for even a few moments, and occasionally when I was with a patient or colleague I was personally close to, and who I knew would not only understand but want to share my grief. A surge of emotion would surface the dozens of times a day I thought of Zach, or when something reminded me of him. I took care, for example, not to glance toward the large westerly window of our 10th floor hospital conference room, with its unimpeded view of the Rocky Mountains, which Zach, a professional pilot, saw every day as he took off in the morning and banked west, and saw again upon returning in the evening accompanied by a majestic sunset or a star-filled sky with a full or partial moon. On one occasion, sitting in the echo reading room and waiting an extraordinarily long time for a study to load on the computer, with a young colleague in the seat next to me—herself pregnant with her first child—I thought out loud, "If this thing doesn't come up soon, I'm going to cry." It didn't, I did, and I then felt a soft, warm hand massaging my slumped and quivering shoulder.

Should I have returned to work so soon? I believe there is no generalizable or correct answer to this question. Our family has learned that individuals grieve in different ways, with each form of grief acceptable to the others. I believe that such individuality is true of a return to work as well. Every loss is different, each loss is felt personally, jobs are different—including the degree of support from colleagues, from which I benefited greatly, and the opportunity for private time during the workday. I returned to work after I was able to control my emotions when it was in the best interest of others to do so. Waiting to return until the raw tenderness of my sorrow lessened would have meant

staying out for months. As bad as I felt, I never thought that griev-
ing impeded my work; if it did, I would have taken it as a sign I had
returned too soon.

My return to work was not all tears and sadness. Having meaningful
work to do took me away for a time from preoccupying thoughts about
what had happened and how I felt. Because medicine by its nature
surrounds us with others who are concerned and caring, I felt much
support from co-workers I met during the day—many of whom had
tears of their own at our first meeting following the accident. Concern
and support often included that offered by patients, and the actions of
two elderly patients are among the most vivid and touching memories
of my return to work.

Ten days after Zach's accident my nurse called me at home saying
that an elderly and long time patient of mine was having problems
and needed to be seen. She asked if I could come over to see him
later that day. I agreed to do so. When I entered his examination room
I witnessed one of the most memorable scenes of my life. He rose
from his chair to greet me and I saw in full how he was clothed: black
shirt, black belt, black pants, black socks, black shoes. There he stood,
expressing his sympathy and mourning for Zach in the old-fashioned
way. His clinical issues were straightforward and readily addressed. He
wanted to see me, but I wondered if this gentle soul wanted most to see
for himself that I was okay, and to tell me face-to-face how sorry he was
about what had happened to our family.

Several days later the second elder was admitted to our coronary
care unit with cardiac, renal, and respiratory failure. As with the first,
I had become friends with him and his family, and his wife and daughter joined us in his room one day during morning rounds. He was
drowsy and barely able to be up in a chair. The vision of him when I
entered his room was in complete contrast to the first patient: I saw
him all in white. He had silver hair, pale skin, and was wrapped in
layers of white blankets. I began to address his clinical issues, wondering if he was alert enough to follow what I was saying. As I spoke, with
effort he raised his head, fixed his pale blue eyes on mine, and said
just above a whisper, "I'm sorry about your son." Exhausted, short of
breath, and barely able to maintain an upright posture, his concern in

that moment was for me. I was moved to tears by his kindness, his wife and daughter wept as well—for all of us, I think—and I thanked him. Several days later he was gone, his multiple organ failure no longer able to support life. One of his last conscious acts was a selfless expression of grief to another ailing soul. It was typical of him, and is a wonderful memory of him.

While there have been countless benevolent acts by others that have provided our family comfort since Zach's death, there is only one thing that has offered any substantial relief to my wife and me. That is illustrated by something that took place on a quiet street in Breckenridge, Colorado, one cold night last December. Those in our family who could make it there had decided to spend a few nights at a lodge outside Breckenridge just before Christmas. One evening we went into town to have dinner in a lovely French restaurant. Zach, who had been giving flying lessons that day in Denver, was to drive up to join us. We kept in touch with him by cell phone as he approached the town, and directed him toward the restaurant. As he neared, I got up and stepped outside to wait for him.

There was no practical reason for me to be standing there, coatless and cold, to help someone find a French restaurant in a small town who could by himself make his way across the country in the dark of night flying a plane thousands of feet in the air. But it was not for practical reasons that I stood there. It was because I was his father. It was to wave to him as his car approached, to welcome him as he walked toward me, to bring him inside where in the warmth and glow of the place he would join his family, joyful at the sight of him, elated that he had come and had arrived safely. My wife only recently recalled a thought she had that evening as we enjoyed each other's company in that lovely place. She remembers sitting back at one point and thinking, "I am totally happy." Three weeks later sorrow caught us.

My stepping outside was a thoughtful thing to do that took no thought to do. It was one of a thousand things we'd done and said of late that made Zach know how he was loved. It is only our certainty of his knowing, which he would have felt deep in his soul even at the moment he lost his life, that provides us a measure of enduring relief. My wife and I agree there was nothing left unexpressed to Zach about our love for him, no regrets about the state of our relationship when he left us. We are free in that regard. Equally important, he was, too.

I have no advice to offer; only a story difficult to share but which I hope may be of help. The new life-clock has ticked off eight months since I took the call on the hallway phone. Sorrow remains, now felt more as a mantle to be borne than tears to be so often shed. Others who have suffered the loss of one so dear tell me the burden lifts with time. I believe that is true, and the mantle is perceptibly lighter than a few months ago. Love being what it is, I know the mantle will be with me always. Love being what it is, I do not object.

In the meantime, we live, as fully as we can. I am buoyed by the presence of a loving family and a generous community of friends and loved ones. I am sustained by having important work to do in the service of others. I am grateful for my life.

Still, I miss him so.

**Dedication:**

For *Monsieur Pilote*, whom we lost, whom we love, and without whom we must learn to travel on, wounded and incomplete.

For any reader who has suffered the loss of one so dear. Only you know the journey beyond imagining. I offer you my deepest sympathy and respect.

To any reader for whom these words might provide comfort, or avoid regret, should such a loss occur.[13]

-------

[13] Hergott L. A Journey Beyond Imagining. *JAMA*. 2009;302(20):2188–2189.

# THE TEARDROP APPROACH

Stop!
Stop it!
Stop what you're doing,
completely.

Listen to me.

This could happen to you.
Don't think you're protected—
we were flourishing before.

Perhaps not this, exactly,
what happened to us,
but This,
yes, it's a definite possibility.

Out of the blue, This
can drop you to your knees
time and again,
your forehead on the floor
like a devout Muslim at prayer—
but you convulsing
in a way only sobbing brings.

It happened to us
on what they call a teardrop approach—
the plane is passing near where it's going to land,
but heading in the opposite direction;

they fly it in a long, wide loop
in the shape of a teardrop
until the plane is back near the starting point
and lined up with the runway.

But our son's plane never made it to the runway.

Country people at their early morning routines
saw the plane come out of the clouds,
low, but "flat and level"—
and then,
suddenly,
it pitched straight down,
and deep into the ground.

The three lost,
all professional pilots,
knew they were on a teardrop approach.
Those of us at home
in the midst of our early morning routines
had no idea that we were, too.

But, then, the call.
And the real teardrops came.
And the hole carved in the ground
was carved in our hearts
to remain,
his presence and absence ever with us.

Flight plans
don't call those traveling
*Souls on Board* for nothing.

What could take a dear one from you
might come suddenly, too—

an impact from a passing car,
a clot in a coronary artery,
a slip on the ice.

But, that thing
that obliterates your concept of what life is
could just as well
proceed slowly—
a mutated cell line, perhaps,
a scrambled brain,
a prelude to a divorce.

Whatever the incident,
the expressed sympathy and good wishes of others,
the size of the crowd at the memorial service,
the smell of blooming lilacs,
Beethoven,
time,
all offer comfort—
but little, in fact,
considering.

Pardon my tapping you on the shoulder
and interrupting whatever it was you were doing.
I don't presume to offer advice.

I only wanted you to know—
that the thing
of consequence to us now,
the thing that matters most,
that offers not just consolation
but a measure of enduring relief,
is our certainty
that,
at that moment,

he knew,
deeply—
from a thousand things we'd done and said
of late—
how we love him.

I thought you'd want to know.[14]

--------

[14] Hergott L. The Teardrop Approach. *Annals of Internal Medicine* 2009;151:753.

# A SEPARATE SACRIFICE

The dimly lit hospital corridor
looks at dusk as it did at dawn.
The patient list in hand, though,
appears much different in the evening light:
names, numbers, tasks—
added, underlined,
crossed off, moved—
cryptic symbols of a day's noble work done
and not yet done.

Moving to the next bedside,
weary,
committed,
sacrificial mantle felt,
I glance toward a westerly window
and am uncaring
to be unmoved
by the known-rapturous palette
of an evening's fleeting majesty—
my soul obscured
until long after duty and privilege are discharged,
the list is satisfied,
and its servant late away.

My beloved's greeting kindles
any time of day
or night.
Food can be rewarmed.

But a day's excited story from a child
now asleep,
told by another,
is absent what could have been eternal between us—
a separate sacrifice
that saddens the most noble heart.[15]

———

[15] Hergott L. A Separate Sacrifice. *Annals of Internal Medicine* 2007;147(12):896.

# COMFORTING A DYING GAUL

On a cloudy winter night in the vast landscape of the St. Benedict Trappist Monastery high in the Colorado Rockies there is blackness everywhere except for two dim lights bordering the monastery's small parking lot. No matter where you are otherwise on the property the sky is black, the land is black, and you can't tell where one stops and the other begins.

On a clear winter night in that landscape there is mostly blackness as well, except for the stars in the sky and the pre-dawn presence of millions of distant, glowing, punctate images you have probably never seen before.

On a sunny winter day two colors dominate—the vivid royal blue sky, and the brilliant white of the snow that covers the ground, including the entirety of the 13,000-foot massif, Mount Sopris—the base of which is on the monastery grounds. The only other things seen in the vast countryside on a sunny winter day are the brilliant golden sun, the small monastery building, and a few dwellings on the side of a hill where retreatants stay.

Excluding the rare sound of an occasional car passing on the small country road, the infrequent spoken words of the monks, and the limited speech of the retreatants, all is quiet except for the occasional rush of a mountain wind. Being in the valley at any time engenders a sense of tranquility and wonder unlike what most of us feel in our daily lives—which is one reason why the retreatants are there, of course.

The monastery's land is so vast and remote there is no mobile phone or internet coverage in the area. A drive several miles into surrounding farmland is required to use a phone. It was upon returning on such a drive one sunny winter afternoon that a physician-retreatant had an unexpected opportunity to manifest the soul of medicine.

The doctor drove carefully coming back over those miles and onto the monastery's narrow, unpaved road. If there had been even a small recent snowfall, it was difficult to tell the difference between the road and a ditch on either side. The day before, she had miscalculated, and her car had suddenly slid toward and then pitched into a ditch, leaving the car at a threatening, snowbound angle. With considerable effort she was able to exit the passenger side of the car, grateful that in doing so she hadn't caused the car to tilt further.

Amazingly, as she stood by the car wondering how she was going to get it out of the ditch a cheerful monk came by driving an enormous snowplow. The monk offered to pull the car out with his snowplow, and as he connected a heavy, clinking chain to a hook under the car's rear fender the monk told the doctor to get in the car, make sure the shift was in the neutral position, and stay there to keep the wheels straight as the snowplow pulled it out of the ditch. Intuiting that the monk had pulled many a car out of a ditch, but still having some apprehension about the mechanics of such an extraction with her in the car, the doctor asked, "Is it possible that the car will roll over as you pull it out?" The monk confidently said, "It's not going to roll over. We do this dozens of times in the winter. Just get in the car, make sure it is in neutral, and keep the wheels straight." Seconds later the car was out of the ditch and upright. The doctor offered a relieved, "Thank you," as the monk waved and drove his massive machine down the hill.

Having risen at 4:00 a.m., which she and others did every morning during the 10-day nondenominational silent retreat, upon returning to the monastery grounds she felt tired and looked forward to taking a nap before the next meditative session. As she turned a curve heading up a hill the doctor saw something troubling in the distant middle of the road. She thought it was an animal that had been hit by a car, but as she approached she saw an elderly man laid out on his side, propped up on one elbow like the marble sculpture, *The Dying Gaul*. The man waved weakly but almost constantly with his free arm, apparently to make certain the driver saw him in the middle of the road. As she got closer the doctor noted small pools of red-tainted snow beneath and around the fallen man, which heightened her concern about why he was lying on the ground.

The doctor recognized the man as one of the retreatants. Knowing little about him, the doctor did recall the man's sadly saying on the first evening of the retreat that he had been diagnosed with disseminated, terminal kidney cancer. He had also despondently shared that his wife died a few months before from a fall and intracranial bleed.

Although a long-time practicing medical subspecialist, the doctor had been a general practitioner in her early years, and her general training surfaced so she could assess the man on the ground. She introduced herself, told him she was a cardiologist, and began the questioning and observations physicians do.

The fallen man was alert. He spoke clearly, and said he had slipped and fallen, and was unable to crawl to the side of the road. When asked, he responded that he did not lose consciousness from the fall, and that his vision was clear. He did not have a headache. He did have several abrasions on his face, and a large bruise on his nose, with blood dripping from his nose. There were abrasions on the palms of his hands and forearms, indicating that on falling to the ground he tried to break the fall, but fell forcefully and face-first on the road.

Though his nose was damaged, there was no focal pain, nor an alteration of the natural structure of his nose—both of which indicated that it was bruised but probably not broken. The doctor took out a tissue and gently compressed the man's nose for the few minutes it took to stop his nosebleed.

The man declined the doctor's offer to call for an ambulance once they would get to the retreat house, where they could use the single landline phone on the property. He said he had been in so many emergency rooms over the past several months he didn't want to go to another, especially considering his prognosis.

After a few minutes, the man was able to stand up with help, walk the few feet to the car with assistance, and get in the front passenger seat. He did well on the short trip to the retreat house. Since it was afternoon silent time there was no one outside or inside the retreat house to help. With the doctor's help the man was able to enter the building and walk slowly to his room. Throughout the time from finding him on the road to getting him to his room the doctor was attentive for the appearance of dizziness, chest discomfort, or shortness of breath. There was none. The doctor helped him lie down on his bed. She found some clean cotton cloths in the man's apartment bathroom, and used them to gently cleanse and dress the bruises.

Though not observing any threatening symptoms or findings, the doctor knew she had nothing more than observation to go on—absent such things as x-rays, blood work, and the expertise of an emergency room physician—and wondered if she was doing the right thing by simply observing the man. She told him there could be an important internal injury that might not be identified by observation, and asked again if he thought he should go to an emergency room. The man ardently denied going there, saying that back home he had told his doctor and his family that he did not want to be resuscitated if his heart stopped. The doctor's medical training told her to send the man to the emergency room, but her medical intuition told her more strongly to honor his decision not to go there.

The man seemed comfortable as he rested quietly on his bed, his affect pleasant but flat, his eyes gazing straight ahead, his face fixed and conveying the sorrowful burden of the loss of his wife, his terminal illness—and now a traumatic fall. He seemed stable, and the doctor no longer had to be as assiduous as she was when she found the man. She had kindly and expertly done what any caring medical practitioner would do. The necessity of emergent care being over, the doctor's fatigue noticeably surged, and she craved rest. She knew that other retreatants could watch over the man safely for a time with minimal directions from her, but there were still none accessible. Thinking the man was probably stable, the doctor considered leaving him to go find someone who could watch him while she rested. It was something beyond thinking, though, that caused her to do what she did next—an act most touching.

Typical of her, completely focused on her new patient's well-being, she set her own weariness aside, and decided not to leave. Staying, she could have sat in comfort and silence anywhere in the room to continue her observation—which was all the man needed physically.

Rather, understanding the patient's needs far beyond the biomedical, the doctor picked up a metal-framed kitchen table chair and placed it next to her patient's bed. Sitting at his bedside, facing him, the doctor leaned forward and tenderly asked, "Tell me about your wife."

-------

# THE MUSCLE MAN

They came into the room one by one as if they were standing in line outside the door, eager to enter and be of service to the young woman soon to undergo complex abdominal surgery.

The surgeon came first—pleased to see her, unpretentiously radiating competence he had earned long ago and kept, consoling her and pledging that the procedure would go well.

The nurse came next—cheerful, comforting, assuring the patient she would be with her the entire time, asking if there was anything at all she could do to make her patient comfortable.

The anesthesiologist followed—her state of being immediately conveying a connection, exuding experience and proficiency. Having recognized subtle anxiety in the patient's demeanor, she assured the patient that she would be given a sedative before leaving her room; and, assured that she, too, would be present during her entire operation, and until she woke up.

Attentively observing what each member of the surgical team said and otherwise expressed, I was heartened about the care my friend was and would be getting. The team members' caring attitude made it clear that, in addition to the concern and attention they would offer, there was a pervasive sense of goodness in them.

The last person to enter the room—and the one most memorable— was the man who would be standing across the operating table from the surgeon, assisting him with the complex technical aspects of the procedure. In about his late-30's, he was large, athletic-appearing, and confident, with a manner of speech bordering on being cocky—a man who knows his business and knows he knows his business.

He went over the technical aspects of the procedure completely, in ways the patient could understand—and made certain after he spoke that she did understand.

As he began to walk toward the door those of us in the room thanked him. Without turning around he loudly said, "You're welcome."

When he got to the door he stopped, turned around, and said something patients and their loved ones rarely hear, but which demonstrates one of the highest forms in the state of being in medicine. "It's a privilege," he softly said, and then turned and left.

———————

# A SMALL, SACRED SPACE

When the staples come out,
and the bone beneath has healed,
and your flowing hair—
artfully parted during—
covers the scar after,
there will be nothing seen
of what proceeded.

If the silken movements
of your Persian surgeon's hands
are allowed to do
what they crave to do,
you will wake up
to no important difference
between who you are
and who you are.

You will recognize you.

But,
as you fear,
if the misplaced membrane
in that small, sacred space
cannot yield
at this chiasm of your life,
and tragedy attempts to insinuate itself,
you may be different.

My most fervent wish
is to assure your normalcy
after.

I cannot.

I can assure you
that those of us who love you now
will long to love
and be loved by you
then—
no matter what.

You will not be alone.

You will not be apart.

Me?
I want to feel again your adoring smile—
one way or the other.

For R.E.S.[16]

--------

[16] Hergott L. A Small, Sacred Space. *Ad Libitum, Annals of Internal Medicine.* 2016; 165(10):752.

# WHAT SHE SAW

It is sometimes an expression of affirmation and gratitude we receive from those we are helping that can amaze and sustain us. One of the most moving affirmations I have received in my career occurred when I wasn't even with the patient.

A young partner of mine, while signing a patient back to me on a Monday morning meeting after I had been off on the weekend, told a joke regarding something the patient said about me after he introduced himself and told her he was covering for me that weekend. "Oh, that doctor," the patient said about me. "He is so good looking."

The joke was not about whether or not I was good looking. The joke was about the large sign her nurses had placed on the wall over the patient's head—stating in large, red letters, *Patient Is Blind*.

My partner found humor in what the patient said, thinking that only someone in her condition could find me attractive. Her statement offered something much more profound, of course, and I was deeply moved by what her comment signified—the cherished connection she and I had made far beyond the physical.

--------

# LOVINGLY CARRIED
# IN A MOTHER'S ARMS

As I came to the end of making rounds in my small-town hospital late one Saturday afternoon long ago I heard the sound of a loud, rustling walk in the distance. Looking toward the sound an alarming vision appeared. In silhouette was a woman frantically rushing down the hallway, holding a young child in her arms. The young woman hollered as she hurried toward some nurses and me that her son was choking from having inhaled a small plastic toy. The boy was coughing vigorously, and as she approached it became clear that he was flaccid in her arms.

I quickly took the child from his mother and laid him on his back on an examination table. His mother stepped back but stayed in the room, to which I did not object. Having heard his cough and the brief story of what had happened, I didn't need to examine the child. I immediately asked the attending nurse to hand me a laryngoscope—a handheld metal device the size of a flashlight that has an extended narrow arm with a small light bulb at its tip—which can be inserted into a patient's mouth to access the airway. Except for coughing frequently the boy was remarkably still as he lay on the table, suggesting that he might be losing consciousness from his inadequate respirations—which made the urgency of extracting the toy even greater.

Standing just above his head at the end of the table, I bent over and gently opened his mouth with my right hand. With my left hand I inserted the arm of the laryngoscope into his mouth, and moved its tip slowly and carefully toward his airway—making certain to open but not damage the epiglottis, a protective flap that opens and closes the airway and rests just above the vocal cords—and guiding the laryngoscope carefully as well to avoid passing it into the esophagus, the orifice of which lies next to the airway orifice and can be misidentified as the airway tube.

The child's coughing increased with the passing of the laryngoscope, which made it harder to identify the vocal cords—likely to be where the toy settled. Moving the device gently forward the light shined on a small, flat red piece of plastic caught between the two cords—nearly filling the space even when the cords were opened to let air through, and not allowing them to close when they were supposed to. Securing the position of the laryngoscope with my left hand held against the child's face, my eyes fixed on the cords, I moved my right hand toward the nurse and asked for a clamp—a device the size and appearance of a small scissors but with two thin blunt metal fingers instead of blades. I felt the clamp placed in my hand and as I began to move it toward the cords a thought flashed in my mind: if in trying to grasp the toy I accidentally displace it downward and beyond the vocal cords, I could completely occlude his airway—which would be catastrophic.

Moving the clamp toward the toy unflinchingly—finding no reason to make things worse by worrying about a failure—I was able to secure the toy in the fingers of the clamp and slowly draw it out of his vocal cords, past the epiglottis, and out of his mouth. The boy coughed deeply a few times after the toy's removal, but the frequency of his coughing quickly decreased, and he seemed to breathe normally between coughs. The nurse and I sat him up and held him briefly on the side of the exam table as I listened to his normal breath sounds with my stethoscope. The nurse then passed the child into his mother's arms.

It was over. He was well.

My memory of those few minutes is vivid, though the incident occurred over forty years ago. I see clearly the small red toy sitting between the boy's vocal cords, and see as well the grip on the toy as I closed the fingers of the clamp. I envision the toy remaining secured as it was gently moved away from the airway.

The most vivid and touching visions though are the contrasting images I saw of how the young mother carried her son toward us, and how she walked as she carried him away; the vision of her frantic, hurried gate as she approached, and of the slow, carefree, graceful way she moved on their way down the hall—her son enfolded in her arms, her head bent with her face close to his, she speaking softly to him in a way no one else could. Able now to reminisce about the event, I feel that the way she cared for him at both times was beautiful. She was doing what caring mothers do, ceaselessly, to express the love they have for their child, in danger or not.

I don't think I reflected in depth at the time about what had happened. I 'simply' did what I needed to do to help the child, felt glad the extraction was successful, and then moved on. Looking back in a deeper way now I see that there is much more history and meaning to the incident: more than a decade of schooling that allowed me to know immediately what I needed to do, and then doing it; my being able to move the clamp without flinching due to training that gave me the confidence to do so; gratitude for the nurse, who helped much more than by simply handing me instruments—her comforting the child, passing her fingers gently through his hair and speaking softly to him as we proceeded, serving as surrogate aunt to him, with his being otherwise in the hands of a large, strange man doing strange things to him.

Reflecting on that critical, successful event now from a distance, perhaps the deepest lesson learned is the awareness that, ultimately, whether specialist or generalist, doctor or nurse, physician assistant or nurse practitioner, pharmacist or administrator, helping patients and their loved ones in need is an *enormous privilege*.

--------

There is an exaggerated but implicative saying in medicine that describes the difference between a generalist and a specialist. A specialist is one who knows everything about something, and a generalist is one who knows something about everything. I was a generalist for a short time early in my career—what in those days was called a General Practitioner and now referred to as a Family Medicine Doctor. It was in those few years that the memorable story of the child in distress took place.

Thinking about it from then to now, as a specialist, I am reminded of how much respect I carry for primary care physicians—pediatricians, family medicine and internal medicine doctors—grateful for their expertise and especially for their outpouring of concern to dig deeply into patients' needs, often at their own cost of time and energy, and thus manifesting the soul of medicine in this very troubling time.

———————

# SOLACE IN LINE AT THE NEIGHBORHOOD COFFEE HOUSE

I couldn't see her face.

I couldn't see the child.

I saw a woman standing in front of me
in line at the neighborhood coffee house
holding a baby.

She looked down
at her baby's face,
and began to sway—
side to side,
gracefully,
unabashedly,

keeping silent time
minute
after minute
after minute.

Perhaps others in the coffee house saw something
cute,
charming.

For me,
the loving unity I perceived
as she held her child
and swayed
meant much more.

I felt within
a quickening sense of light and warmth—
knowing from that moment that
there is hope for the Earth.

———

# NOEL

The clearest example I can offer of subjectivity being aligned with the essence of medical practice also comprises the most precious compliment I have received as a doctor. The incident occurred during an office visit with a patient.

Noel is an evangelical Christian preacher of a small congregation. As such, he often cites scripture or Christian tenets during our visits. He knows from my non-responsive responses that I do not share his belief system, but neither am I hostile to it. Our meetings have always been cordial.

At one of our visits Noel sadly said that his wife of many years had died two weeks earlier. She had suffered a cardiac arrest in their home, had undergone a prolonged resuscitation there, and died a few hours later in a hospital emergency room.

Several days after her death Noel went to her doctor's office to learn more about the specifics of her health issues and her death. Noel's wife had mentioned to him that she did not feel close to her doctor, that their visits were businesslike, and her doctor's demeanor distant. After hearing what his wife's physician had to say, Noel told the man, "I don't know why you didn't treat her the way my doctor treats me. I don't actually know what my doctor thinks of me personally, but I think he loves me."

# JUST THE RIGHT WORDS

"I love you," the woman said to the cardiologist
as he turned and walked toward his computer
at the end of their consultation.

Having never heard a patient say that—
and not knowing whether she was joking or not—
he said nothing,
and waited for what he hoped would be a chuckle,
and a remark that she meant he had done a very good job.

A moment later, though, she said again, "I love you,"
and after a pause added sincerely,
"I have fallen in love with you."

He wondered hastily about what words he should use
to tell her that because of what she said
he would no longer be her cardiologist,
nor ever see her again.

As the cardiologist turned to say the required words she
spoke again.
"But, I suppose you get that a lot," she said in a tone either
disappointed
or in a forced attempt at humor.

As the cardiologist started to say what he had planned to
say—

to not only let her know they would never see each other
again,
but also not to embarrass or debase her—
the planned words disappeared,
and from some silent somewhere he jested,
"You know, even from the men!"

Any tension in the room vanished.

The cardiac work was done.

The patient's inappropriate statement was addressed and
understood.

The doctor did not shame her.

Any sense of fault was hers to ponder.

The twice-startled cardiologist grateful for the wellspring of
creativity that sprung the placating reply.

------

# SOLITARY MAN

When I enter the examination room in which a new patient sits, often accompanied by one or more loved ones, I sense two questions on their faces: *Does he know? Does he care?* Is he well trained, and an expert? Has he kept up with medical literature and treatments? Will he care about how I feel, or what I fear? Will he be concerned about, and respect, those with me? Will he take the time needed to address what matters to me physically and otherwise?

Hopefully, within about ten minutes of our being together their questions are answered in the affirmative. Sensing their relief—from the changes in their faces, posture, and verbal tone—I can then proceed without concern about reservations they may have had, and open the trove of knowledge I can access to help them. A memorable experience I had with a newly hospitalized man demonstrates the good that can ensue between a doctor and a respectful but questioning patient.

The first time I entered his hospital room I felt there was something exceptional about him. In his mid-60's with no previous health problems, he had been admitted to the hospital with chest pain the day before, and was thus assigned to my cardiology team to determine if his chest discomfort was coming from a blocked coronary artery, inflammation of the sack-like tissue that covers the heart called the pericardium, or from some other cardiac or chest malady. He greeted me in a reserved but not unpleasant manner. As we conversed I felt that he was gauging me intensely. Neither his demeanor nor his chest symptoms, though, were what seemed exceptional about him. Rather, it was the small stack of well-read books on his bedside table that seemed remarkable.

As I asked about his medical and personal histories he was respectful but succinct in his responses. His social history revealed that he was a single man with no children. He lived alone. His work was the repairing of damaged furniture. I asked if he carved or built furniture and he said he did not. Though he seemed intelligent and scholarly, his was manual labor.

After taking his histories and doing an examination I explained what I would like to do to clarify the cause and relevance of his symptoms. I then answered the thoughtful questions he asked. As our conversation progressed his affect seemed less stiff, as did his posture as he sat in a chair at the side of his bed, his books on the portable table in front of him. Later in the day as I shared more test results and made further recommendations, he seemed to drop any reservations he had about me. By the end of the day, it seemed that our conversation was as casual as two friends visiting.

The results of the x-rays, CT scans, and laboratory tests revealed that his was not a cardiac condition. To the disappointment of us all, he was found to have cancer that was disseminated so diffusely in his body that we could not identify the original site of the malignancy. The cell type was adenocarcinoma, not uncommonly known to present late in its course, and thus with diffuse metastases.

He took the news of the diagnosis without overt emotion. I knew he took it seriously but, as was his nature, his subjective thoughts and feelings were left his own. As expected, he asked several questions about treatments and prognosis. I explained that, due to his diagnosis being cancer rather than a cardiac condition, he would be transferred to the oncology team, and that they would go over treatments and prognosis in detail. He then said, "Cancer throughout the body must have a poor prognosis." Though our interactions were short I felt that he considered me to be a counselor, and I was willing to serve as such up to the level of my general medical knowledge. I had many patients and friends with widely disseminated adenocarcinoma. "The prognosis is poor," I said. "In such a case chemotherapy can slow the progress of the malignancy, but the chance of cure is not good." He thanked me for my response and obvious concern. The transfer to the oncology team was made that afternoon. My clinical responsibilities were over. The discussion he had with the senior oncologist regarding prognosis was essentially the same as the one we had.

Though he was no longer my patient formally, in another way I felt that he still was and I visited him in his hospital room on occasion. When I entered his room on my first visit with him after his transfer I mentioned that another patient of mine, a 44-year-old woman, had just received the same diagnosis as his. He asked if she had a family and I told him she had a husband and two young children—that both of us knew she would soon leave behind. Hearing so brought tears to his eyes. He shared that his tears reflected empathy for her, but he added tenderly that he was also moved to know that in his condition he could feel such empathy.

Late in the afternoon a few days later I realized that I hadn't visited with him in a while. I called the Oncology floor and asked if he was still there. An Oncology nurse told me he was but that he was to be discharged to home the next morning, a Saturday. She said that no chemotherapy treatment was to be administered. He was to be sent home with palliative care.

I wanted to see him before he left, but it was into the early evening that I learned of his incipient discharge—and my wife, Diane, and I had a dinner party to go to. I asked Diane if it would be all right with her if on our way to the party I paid a visit to a terminal patient who was to be discharged the next morning. As is her nature, she not only said it would be fine to do so, but she sat in the car outside the hospital waiting in a mild rain for the 30 minutes I spent with him.

Our visit had a sense of gravity. He knew he was close to death, and said a few things about his life and how he felt about dying. My job was to listen, of course, not as a physician this time, but as a friend. He said, "I fear death," but then immediately followed with an unforgettable, corrective statement, "No," he said, "I loathe death. I fear being cared for by someone who wouldn't drop by at 6:00 o'clock on a Friday evening."

I shared the visit with Diane. She, too, was moved by the visit, and knew it was good for both my patient and me.

He left the hospital the next day. I never saw him again.

For me, the brief time we were together over those few days was an inspiring, life-learning experience. He was profound. He was a sage. He taught me about how meaningful the briefest of comments can be.

He taught me what it can be like to face death and still have a sense of otherness. He was alone, but held knowledge about others—perhaps especially from the books he had at home and which he brought to the hospital. He knew he was soon to die, yet had wept upon learning that someone else was also to die, and leave her young family absent her presence forever. He had the temperament to weep knowing that even in his state he could be empathetic to the tragedy of a stranger. In the colossal implications of his terminal state he was moved and comforted by the simple gesture of a bedside visit on a rainy Friday night.

Some months later I wrote an essay titled *Playing the Moonlight Sonata From Memory: Celebrating the Wonders of Our Difficult Life*. The essay discusses the harm and devastation we may cause patients and their loved one in our practices, but asks readers to remember as well the many wonders of medicine. Experiencing my cancer patient was a wonder of medicine. Grateful for our time together I decided to dedicate the essay to him.

To do so, and thus publish his name in the worldwide *Journal of the American Medical Association (JAMA)*, I had to get permission from relatives who survived him. I found his address and phone number in his medical record. His phone number was no longer operative. I called the man whose phone number was listed as someone to call in an emergency. The person listed turned out to be the patient's landlord, who told me the patient had no family. We had no one to give permission to publish his name. He had been truly alone.

Having fulfilled the obligations necessary, but finding no one to give us permission to do so, the editors at *JAMA* allowed me to proceed. In writing the dedication I felt that I was honoring a friend, and expressing gratitude and respect for him. In as succinct a way as he would have said, I wrote at the end of the essay, "In memory of Charles Hyams."

-------

# I FELT SOMETHING POP
# INSIDE MY HEAD

The handsome young man in suit and tie, accompanied by his equally pleasant wife, said after I asked what had brought him to our emergency room, "I felt something pop inside my head."

My immediate thought upon hearing what he said was that he might have partially ruptured an aneurysm in an artery of his brain—though he had none of the classic symptoms of a ruptured cerebral artery aneurysm: a sudden, severe headache, and loss of consciousness.

I took a full history from him in an attempt to rule in or out other diagnoses that could have caused such a symptom. I heard nothing from his story that pointed to a different diagnosis. His physical examination, including a neurologic examination, was normal. His blood work was normal.

Still suspicious that the young man's symptom indicated a partially ruptured aneurysm I phoned the neurology resident on call, who would be the one treating such a condition, and asked him to come down to the emergency room to consult on the patient. The resident did so with reluctance, unimpressed by my concern. After completing his evaluation he declared that the patient did not have a ruptured aneurysm, and that he would not be performing a lumbar puncture on the patient—the test that in those days would rule in or out my hypothesis. A lumbar puncture showing blood in the cerebrospinal fluid drained would indicate a ruptured aneurysm and lead to an emergent and potentially lifesaving neurosurgical procedure to find and occlude the aneurysm. Deferring to the specialty resident's opinion rather than following my intuition I discharged the patient from the emergency room.

Two weeks later I got a call from a physician at a hospital across town informing me that the young man had come to their emergency room with a severe headache, had suddenly lost consciousness, and died there. An autopsy confirmed a ruptured cerebral artery aneurysm.

I felt terrible upon hearing the news, knowing that even though his presenting symptom was atypical, I had drawn the right conclusion, and thus had a chance to save his life. I thought about the devastating feeling his wife would be experiencing—their anticipated long lovers' journey prematurely ended in an instant. I wondered if the couple had children, dazed and disoriented as they felt for the first time the empty, unnatural absence of their father—a feeling that would be with them forever.

I was a second-year internal medicine resident without direct professorial supervision when I cared for the young man. Now, 40 years later, I still think of him and his wife on occasion. Having experienced deep personal loss myself, I hope the patient's wife and family have been able to live the fullest lives possible—albeit carrying the sorrowful sense of being wounded and incomplete.

Penitently reviewing the course of events that led to the patient's death I reflected on the concept of responsibility. My patient's story is an example of the two types of responsibility physicians and other decision makers face: *absolute* responsibility and *ultimate* responsibility. Absolute responsibility occurs in medicine when the diagnosis and treatment in a case are made by one clinician only. Ultimate responsibility occurs when more than one individual influences decision making, but only one person decides which course of action to take.

It came to me that I was *ultimately* responsible for my patient's death and for his family's devastation. I was ultimately responsible because it was I who made the decision to accept the "expert opinion" of the neurology resident, thus change my diagnostic plan, and discharge the patient from the emergency department—eliminating any chance for a correct diagnosis and successful treatment.

Was the neurologist partially responsible for the patient's death because his opinion altered my plan? Yes, he missed the diagnosis, but, no, there is no *partial* responsibility. *I* was in charge of the case, *I* asked for and accepted the consultant's advice, and *I* decided to let my patient go. Another party's input or not, I made the ultimate decision—which is why it's called *ultimate* responsibility.

---

# WHAT I LEARNED
# FROM JOHN DENVER

The arrival of a letter notifying me of an *Emeritus Professor of Medicine* designation was not unexpected. Someone present at the meeting informed me that a University of Colorado committee had voted unanimously in favor of bestowing the title upon my retirement. Unexpected was what accompanied the letter—a deluge of vivid reminiscences of personal and academic troubles I had in my training years that would have made such a designation unimaginable.

I struggled inordinately from my first day in medical school well into my internal medicine residency, not just because of the gargantuan amount of information others and I needed to learn over those years but from a mystifying, pervasive feeling of being inept and overwhelmed. Feeling overwhelmed in medical school was not and is not exceptional, especially in the first few months. My state of shock lasted much longer than the first few months. Even understanding how exceptional it was that, having played two varsity sports in college, I was accepted into medical school a year early did not reassure me that I belonged there.

The word *overwhelmed* doesn't come near describing how I felt. I felt a chaotic, sustained, disorienting, desolate emotional paresis. I was in an unfathomable world. I did not recognize myself. I skipped gross anatomy dissection labs almost every session of the second semester. I took some bad advice from another medical student—who said I didn't need to go to the Embryology class lectures to pass the course, but only review the textbook the weekend before the final exam. I reviewed the textbook but, having *no* idea what the questions in the test were about, I flunked Embryology. I am certain that my first-year medical school troubles placed me deep into the lower 10% of my class at the end of the year.

I persevered, and as my training years progressed, which included starting an internal medicine residency at the University of California-Davis, my sense of self improved, as did my academic and clinical performance. But, that progression continued to be accompanied by oppressive feelings of self-doubt and, as clinical responsibilities increased, worry that I could do harm to patients.

The lowest of the low points came in the middle of my first year of internal medicine residency, when I had a crisis of confidence so severe that, fearing I would do harm to hospitalized patients assigned to me, I had to leave work—on my first 24-hour shift as the admitting medical resident at my hospital. A colleague generously agreed to cover for me and, with the concerned consent of the head of the residency program, I left to spend a melancholy and bewildering day at home. The day after that darkest of days I returned to work and declined the director's offer to arrange a visit with a psychiatrist for me. I recall upon my return being embarrassed that my co-residents and others knew what had happened but, far more, I was relieved that I had not done harm that day. I continued to plod along in the residency, but four months after the day I had to leave work I started a rotation that unexpectedly pulled me out of the deep pit in which I had dwelled for so long, and changed *everything*—a transformation facilitated in part by the music of John Denver.

That year of residency ended with a two-month emergency room rotation during which I oversaw, effectively without faculty guidance, all internal medicine cases while alternating 12-hour day and night shifts weekly with another resident. The night shifts were especially difficult due to the need to handle a high volume of cases with no sleep. I recall falling asleep sitting on the couch more than once while talking to Diane and our three children upon getting home the morning after a shift.

To prepare for the night shifts I took up the habit of lying on our living room floor listening to John Denver's music for a half-hour or so before leaving for work. John's words and music calmed and inspired me. The theme of much of his music was celebratory and hopeful, and emphasized a sense of otherness. His words and music brought joy and meaning to many, but they seemed to especially encourage young men like me (age 29 at the time) to understand that it was all right to feel and share those feelings, to be concerned about families beyond our own, to be concerned about more than our jobs and ourselves, to take a stand and be an outward-looking man. I think the calmness, hope, and otherness the music offered are what helped me most on those night shifts, turning me away from the self-protective traits I had adopted to compensate for my perceived inadequacies, and toward the needs of patients and their loved ones—an opening of the soul of medicine for me.

There were other things that aided my transformation during those two months. I had an increasing awareness of generating sophisticated treatment plans and making correct diagnoses in complex cases—sometimes after others had missed the diagnoses. It is also possible that during the emergency room rotation I had reached a critical point of assimilating enough information and managing enough cases that I could cross the threshold to competence. These and other clinical factors may explain how I came to do *what I did* in patient care, but it was what I learned from John Denver's music and presence that largely influenced *how I felt* about what I did. John's music touched a deep part of me, and guided me toward a path that not only helped change my sense of self, but over time my sense of the world.

At the end of the emergency room rotation I felt competent and confident for the first time—and have never felt otherwise since. My sentence—from whatever source—in a reflexive, pathologic, self-imposed, and very dark prison ended. Most gratifying was my feeling a joyous sense of *liberation*, released from how I had *been* in medicine for so long.

As time passed and my training ended our family moved to Denver, Colorado where I joined a cardiology practice that was not only dedicated to clinical excellence but also to a balanced life. A few years after moving to Colorado—and about ten years after my transformative emergency room rotation—I met John Denver for the first time.

One summer, John, Colorado's then governor Richard Lamm, and others sponsored a concert on the state capitol lawn opposing nuclear weapons. As a board member in one of the sponsoring groups, *Physicians for Social Responsibility/International Physicians for the Prevention of Nuclear War* (which received the 1985 Nobel Peace Prize), I was invited to attend a press conference announcing the event at a church in Denver. A personal interaction with John and my son, Zachary, that morning is one of my favorite memories in life, and offers insight into who John was, why he mattered, and why we trusted him.

The press conference was held in the sanctuary of the church, and some of us were invited to sit on chairs placed alongside the table where John was sitting and answering the press's questions. I had brought Zachary, then about five years old, with me. At a silent moment in the proceedings Zach let out a long, contented, loud sigh. That caused John to look toward us. What he saw was a young boy sitting on his loving father's lap, the child's head resting peacefully on his father's chest. That vision brought a broad, beaming smile to John's face, the image of which I treasure. Zach's eyes must have met John's as well, something I feel good about. After the press conference I introduced Zach to John, who said with an adoring and animated smile, "Hiya, Zach! I have a son named Zach, too."

Diane and I visited with John a few more times during the weeks of the promotion and concert. He was always welcoming, down to earth, and respectful. We treasured the interactions we had with him over that brief period. As the three of us stood chatting after the concert I thought about telling John that at a critical time in my life and career his music helped me in a very crucial way. I decided not to tell him, thinking that doing so would simply seem to him another fan's idolization. As I think of it now, I wish I had told him. I was not idolizing him. I was thanking him, and his sensitivity would have recognized that what was said was not adoration, but rather the telling of a story that because of his work a life was changed that benefitted many other lives.

In the fading stages of John's career some long-standing difficulties in his personal life began to dominate his behavior and define his public persona. He wrote openly of these in his book, *Take Me Home: An Autobiography*. Disillusionment among many of John's admirers, including me, followed as his divorce, short-lived remarriage, and dysfunctional personal habits tarnished his reputation—and his ability to inspire.

Not long before his death I came across John's mother, who lived in Denver, in the lobby of St. Joseph Hospital. We had a lovely chat, though she expressed concern about him over the well-publicized personal difficulties he was having. I told her how much John had meant to my family and me. What I chose not to tell her was that I felt so betrayed by John's behavior I had decided not to spend any more money on his recordings.

Then, we lost him, and another lesson was learned. I thought about just how much his work and (most of) his life had inspired me. I vowed then to not so easily give up on people, a vow I have kept.

Some years after his death John Denver was the first person enshrined in the Colorado Music Hall of Fame. A vibrant but nostalgic concert celebrating his music, performed by members of his band and other well-known musicians, was presented to several thousand fervent fans at the ceremony. The evening ended with a short speech by his first wife, Annie—who had both shared John's climb to superstardom and been subjected to his infidelity and other misbehaviors that finally ended their marriage.

I had some concern about what she would say. Annie shared a few things about their time together and ended her short speech by saying of John, "He was beautiful."

Yes, he was—and so were the many gifts he gave to the world, not the least of which were those given to my family, my patients, and me.

---

# AN ELEVATOR BLESSING

I believe that even in this era of medical care the great majority of clinicians do everything they can for their patients, and honor the call they devoted themselves to when they began to care for them. Doing so, they also remain true to what the late Irish philosopher and poet John O'Donohue counseled in his poem, *For Presence*, "Respond to the call of your gift and the courage to follow its path."

Our path is often brutally hard to follow. We could easily feel at times that we are traveling on a different path, the one mentioned in the opening line of Dante's *Inferno*: "In the middle of the road of my life I awoke in a dark wood where the true way was wholly lost" (Sayers/Reynolds translation).

The persistent curtailing of clinician and patient interaction-times may send us on yet another path, one that leads to the extinguishing of the *soul of medicine—that thing beyond the biomedical, immutable, sustaining: the caring, compassionate, dedicated, enthusiastic attitude that set us on the difficult-by-nature, enriching journey called the medical life.* For understandable but tragic reasons—and not by our choice—the soul of medicine is too often smoldering rather than flaming in the hearts of clinicians. Manifestations of the soul of medicine can occur, though, even in the simplest scene—like an elevator descending, as the coming story tells.

A senior colleague stepped into an elevator car and expressed how pleased he was to be on his way home after a long and wearing day. When the elevator stopped and its doors opened a few floors down no one entered the car until the doors were about to close. Then came the sudden vision of two legs and feet in a wheelchair that was noisily and quickly moving forward as a very elderly woman was being pushed into the car, apparently by her son. The son called to his father, still unseen in the hallway, who finally entered the car slowly and turned to face the door with pronounced dependence on a cane—as the doctor held the button that kept the doors open until everyone was in the car and settled.

The woman in the wheelchair, apparently a patient who had just seen her physician, did not look well. She was pale and much thinner than her body structure indicated. She kept her head down and still, her face fixed in a lifeless gaze toward the back of the car floor. She neither spoke to nor looked toward her son, her husband, or anyone else in the car. She was wearing a purple windbreaker.

From the silence in the car as it began to descend came the doctor's voice, speaking to the woman. "You look like you're dressed to go to the Colorado Rockies game tonight." She did not move, change her stare, or respond. After an uncomfortable silence her son said, "It's a Kansas State University jacket. The Wildcats."

"Oh, the Wildcats," the physician said to the woman. "I saw them play football against the University of Colorado Buffaloes a few years ago. You can't do much better than the Wildcats."

After another long pause, with other passengers coming and going as the elevator stopped and started again, staring straight ahead the woman said in a dreary tone, "I went to school there."

"What did you study there?" the doctor then asked, as the woman's son whispered, "Wow!"—obviously surprised that the physician was taking the time to engage his mother. The son then took a long look at the doctor's badge.

The woman lifted her head and turned toward the doctor. With a flat tone she said, "Laboratory Medicine," adding after another pause, this time in a more animated tone, "Nobody has ever asked me what I studied there."

The physician responded, "Well, I want to thank you for all you did for our patients and us over the years."

The woman tilted her head and focused on the doctor's face for the first time.

"You're welcome," she said softly, continuing her stare. Her son's gaze was fixed on the doctor as well, and both continued that look until they began to leave the elevator.

Starting to exit the car and enter the lobby the woman's son stopped and said, "Thank you, doctor, for talking to my mom."

"My pleasure," said the physician as the family left and the doors closed.

Neither the physician nor anyone else spoke as the car descended one more floor and we all exited to the parking lot. Perhaps those in the elevator were as moved as I by what they had seen.

A physician, tired, eager to be away but sensing consuming distress in a patient of someone else, risked initiating a conversation with her, and affirming her for a life's work in laboratories serving patients and medical staffs she rarely saw. Because of the doctor's attention and kindness, medical and non-medical people present in the car, and especially her son, had the opportunity to see the lightening of her mood and the lessening of her sense of separation.

It was beautiful.

There was a lot to ponder about that brief but moving scene. One thing to conclude was that the physician, though physically drained, was far from having *compassion fatigue*, something increasingly seen in medical practice. The gift of presence the doctor gave to the patient reminded me of something I read in Thomas Merton's book, *Conjectures of a Guilty Bystander*, about a beneficent trait French theologian Francois Fenelon and American Cardinal John Henry Newman seemed to have in common, though they lived in different centuries. They had, wrote Merton, "The same way of looking at you, of listening to you, with a respect you could not imagine you had suddenly deserved."

The physician in the elevator had blessed the woman—and all of those in the car, in a way—exhibiting one definition of the essence of medicine: *All day long, and on many nights, we bless others as the work blesses us.*

Until time passes and the structure of medical care improves, perhaps we should as often as possible try to be in the state-of-giving of the doctor in the elevator—and thus sense, in profound moments of care on our path, the gratifying warmth of the soul of medicine.

———————

# TRAGEDY OF SHADOWS

We'll neither know what shaped your choice,
the thing or things that stopped you.
I cannot know without your voice—
your voice entombed chose not to
say or even glance
at what it was that stilled the dance.[17]

--------

[17] Hergott L. Tragedy of Shadows. *Ad Libitum, Annals of Internal Medicine.* 2015; 163;644.

# THE ABSENCE OF SOMETHING

Having lost interest in the grand rounds lecture being given, I began to glance around the large hall. Patches of sunshine set certain things alight, one of which was a colleague's left hand resting on the table in front of him. My gaze fixed on that image because there was something unnatural in its look, not from a deformity of his hand but from the absence of something—the gold wedding ring I had seen him wear for decades. I had been thinking about him as the first anniversary of his wife's death approached. I wondered how he was doing, when he had removed the ring, and why surviving spouses do.

The act of removing a wedding ring in such a circumstance must be a declaration of some kind. Is a ring's removal a statement to the self, "I no longer feel married," or a statement to the beloved lost, "I will always treasure you, but I must let go"? Intended or not, such an act is a message to the world, "I am no longer married." And, at least for some, "I am no longer married and I am available." A wedding ring's removal could be a sign that the sight or feel of it was too painful a reminder of the presence that was and the absence that is. Glancing at my friend's hand once more, I wondered what the future holds for him. I wondered, too, what absences the future might hold for me, or for those I love.

Our family knows absence. My wife and I abide one of the most devastating kinds of absence, that caused by the death of a child. Our son, Zachary, was killed in a plane crash at 7:00 a.m. on January 15th, 2009. Our family feels his loss most painfully on that date, easily the worst day of the year for us. Every January 15th my wife and I rise early and sit in our living room in darkness except for the glow of a gentle fire. At 6:30 we light a candle and track the course of the 30-minute flight across Colorado that took Zach's life, and mark in deep sorrow the moment we lost him. Then, through tears, with halting speech, we read out loud John O'Donohue's poem, *On the Death of the Beloved*, which lovingly describes Zach in each stanza—as it does others' beloveds lost. The poem's final stanza implies hope for the future, and offers an inspirational way to live on in the presence of encumbering sorrow. We then share stories about Zach, which lessens our sadness and allows us to eventually move to expressions of gratitude for the joy and wonder his presence brought for the 32 years we had him. The ritual bonds the two of us ever more deeply and evokes a sense of immense gratitude in each that we are not alone in the sorrow and joy of living on.

Through stories of loss told by others—from colleagues, friends, and patients to hospital workers I didn't know who approached me in the lunch line—we learned soon after Zach's death that, while the circumstances of our loss are uncommon, our suffering is not extraordinary. Far more people than I would have imagined suffer from deep absences of various kinds. A woman who scans documents into the electronic medical record in our office shared that her infant brother died 20 years before, and that her parents still visit his grave every Sunday. A man in his mid-80's who comes to see me once a year gets tearful when at each visit he describes the death of his 21 year-old son, who was hit by a car thirty years ago, "Only a block from home."

The husband of a recent new patient turned an examination room into a confessional when, with his wife sitting next to him, he said for the first time that he was responsible for the death of their daughter 19 years ago. After his wife had mentioned their daughter's death in a car accident I briefly stared at him because I thought I saw a mist come to his eyes. Noticing my stare, he said, "I was driving the car." After a long pause he added, "I fell asleep." His wife was astonished. "I thought you couldn't remember if you fell asleep," she said. "I fell asleep," he repeated, as more tears came.

The most poignant memory for me of a shared story of absence after Zach's death was one wholly unexpected. I had driven to an automobile garage in our neighborhood to get the title out of Zach's car so we could transfer ownership to his brother. As I left my car and walked toward the garage I saw Zach's car in the work area. Instead of going through the office door I went directly into the work area, opened the glove compartment, took the title out—and then noticed that I had been under the stare of a mechanic standing several yards away. I concluded from his persistent look that I was not supposed to be in that area and walked quickly to my car.

As I looked up after starting the engine I was startled to see the mechanic standing outside my window. I opened the window, expecting to be chastised. Instead, he softly said, "I'm sorry about your son." *I'm sorry about your son*; tender words of sympathy from a total stranger. I got out of the car to thank him and could tell that he was shy, which added even more to his expression of sympathy. Repetitively stroking the work rag he was holding, he then solemnly shared the loss of his eight year-old son years before, who did not survive complex congenital heart disease surgery. Genuinely sad about the death of my son, seeing me brought to the surface the underlying sorrow he carries for the loss of his own.

I later thought, "This man is somebody's patient. I wonder if his doctor knows the emotional burden he carries." That thought affirmed my practice of taking a social history at every patient's first visit, and the importance of knowing who patients are as well as what malady they may have.

Of the many burdens a patient or physician may carry, the death of a beloved is among the worst, but I have learned that there are other kinds of absences individuals may feel similarly. A young friend wrote to tell me after Zach's death that her grief, which began abruptly when her husband announced he no longer wanted to be a husband and father and walked away, was not unlike our grief. She too lost her beloved—totally, unexpectedly, and in an instant. Pondering the similarity of my young friend's sudden loss to ours, I can imagine the opposite—a long prelude to a devastating divorce being akin to the slow, sorrowful leaving of a loved one dying of cancer or a terminal neuromuscular illness. The same could be true of "losing" a loved one still physically present whose personhood has been taken away by dementia or a stroke.

In caring for others we physicians deal with absences, or the threat of them, routinely. Although we are not and should not be paralyzed by the fact, even the most common ailments carry a potentially serious threat to a patient's wellbeing or survival. Some diagnoses we make are seriously threatening to patients and demand extreme treatments from us to prevent disability or death. Others toll the bell for impending, ultimate absence the instant the diagnosis is shared with the patient—and thus direct our care to patient issues beyond the biomedical as well as to the biomedical.

Aging patients often share with physicians troubling limitations from degeneration in mobility, cognition, hearing, sight—ultimately fearing the total loss of any of these. Patients and friends with hearing impairment have told me they feel excluded from a conversation, and thus isolated from those they are with, if they miss even a few words of what is said and thus cannot understand a statement made. Many such people have soberly shared that they miss the enjoyment of music they have treasured all their lives, and no longer attend concerts or even play music in their homes. Several patients have said that impairment of their vision has affected them more personally than chronic pain or other symptoms, having taken away their lifelong joy of reading books, or seeing clearly the faces of people they are with. Women who have had a breast or uterus removed have expressed profound grief especially over the symbolic losses such procedures bring.

In the midst of all we hear from patients, colleagues, friends, or strangers regarding their health concerns or experiences of loss, the fact that they trust us with their personal stories is a gratifying affirmation that we are being of service to them—and exemplifies one definition of the essence of medicine: All day long, and on many nights, we bless others as the work blesses us.

The most vivid image I have of my friend whose wife died a year ago is not that of seeing his left hand absent his wedding ring. The most vivid image is something I saw at her wake: the vision of his head resting softly on the chest of his older brother, whose arm cradled him as they stood together near her open casket. Courageously allowing us to see his vulnerability, my friend gave those present a great gift. The scene told everything anybody who doesn't already know could ever know about the pain of deep, personal absence.

Last night, as I was reading to my three-year-old granddaughter before putting her in the crib—her head resting softly on my chest—she raised her head, gave me a kiss on the cheek, and then laid her head down again. Several weeks ago in the same setting, as I stood over her crib just before her eyes closed she looked up at me and said, "Will you be here when I wake up?" *Will you be here when I wake up. I want you to be here when I wake up. I want you to be with me. I love you, Grandpa.*

I want to be with her, and with all whom I hold dear, including my patients. Intensely aware of the devastating feeling absence can cause—but also of the richness of presence—I will do all I can to delay the absence of something in their lives being the absence of me.[18]

––––––

[18] Hergott L. The Absence of Something. *JAMA*. 2015;313(12):1215–1216.

# REGARDING A LETTER
# TO A DYING FRIEND

Through long hours and too many deaths,
this I have learned:
every word counts now.

Your friend spends his days
consumed by the news.

He needs you.

Choose your words thoughtfully,
and not about you.

Write nothing that derails
or otherwise impairs
the one with little time left.

Write something soon that kindles
your bond.

Thank him for enriching your life,
and for his many affections
compelling you to write to him.

Tell him of your heavy sadness
to learn that the tumor had spread,
that the agonizing treatments had failed.
Manifest respect,

and concern,
never pity.

Tell him how moved you are
by his courage.
Emphasize the obvious in him—
no surprise—
an unremitting sense of
strength,
and grace.

Sing his praises for these.

Send gifts.
His life is not over.
Send yourself.

Give the gift of your presence on his end journey,
declaring that, far away,
you cannot walk with him
but you can walk beside him
in spirit.

Give him the gift of knowing
he matters now and always will,
that with your own immense loss
memories of him
will live in you forever.

When that time comes to say goodbye,
give him the greatest gift,
and tell him you love him.[19]

--------

[19] Hergott L. Regarding a Letter to a Dying Friend. *Ad Libitum, Annals of Internal Medicine.* 2019;170(4):274.

# IN THE NAME OF PRESENCE

My nurse is having a bilateral mastectomy next week—
a preventive procedure offering to prolong her life.

She is paying a steep and intimate price
for what she has decided is an even larger benefit.

Her mind aware in anticipation of her loss,
she is committed to the future—
an imagined, distant place when put next to
what she knows is coming soon. But,

she wants to see her boys become men, and thriving.
She wants to walk hand-in-hand into the ocean with her
grandchildren—
her beloved husband on the beach taking a photo of that
enduring scene.
She wants to love and be loved by him—
long term.

Is she brave, courageous, heroic?

It's not for us to say—
and her concerns are not about a label.

Is she willing to be absent a treasured part of herself now
and forever
in the name of presence then?

Yes.

Well, what is that?
Is that love?

Yes. It is.

That's all it is.

All.

For K.J.C.

-------

# RESTING, CONTENTED, IN A HOUSEHOLD OF BELOVEDS

*"Be kind, for everyone you meet is fighting a great battle."*

– Philo of Alexandria

"Is my wife having an affair?" the wounded voice on the other end of the telephone line asked. The caller, the husband of a colleague, had offered this as his first sentence upon phoning me at home late one evening. He wanted to know where his wife was, and why she was yet again absent from their home as he sat waiting with their young children. Initially stunned by the bluntness of his question, I quickly understood its logic, and knew why he was asking. I also had a good idea of where she probably was and who she was with. Even so, I thought that no matter what I thought, it was not my place to answer such a question. I was about to tell him that he needed to ask it of her when he spoke again. "I know that you value family life, and that you will be honest with me," he sadly said.

We were all friends. Didn't he deserve some kind of response? Perhaps, but any answer tendered to such a question had better be on target and helpful, or unnecessary harm and hard feelings could ensue. Had I seen telltale signs of her having a relationship with another man? It would almost certainly have had to be someone at work, since it was clear that she spent virtually all of her time either there or at home. Had I witnessed recurring, lingering conversations between a co-worker and her, or seen her leaving campus with another man during the day? Had there been episodes of a male nurse, physician, or staff member serving as confidante to her? Knowing her, caring about them both, and feeling that my notion was probably accurate, I risked an answer.

"I don't think your competition is another man," I said. "I think it's work. She is almost certainly at the hospital doing a case. I have never seen her pay any undue attention to another man. I do know the inordinate depth of commitment and sense of mission she holds regarding her work. The only man by her side is probably a nurse handing her instruments." He seemed to take comfort from my response. Yet, we both knew that his relief was partial, and that even though he was probably not caught in a heart wrenching struggle with another man, he still had the formidable rival of work.

We meet few villains in medicine. I can identify no villain in the story just related. There may be victims in such situations, though, especially children, who, while having little role in the decision making about how their parents distribute work and family time, have been known to possess long memories about the effects of such decisions. There is in the story a poignant example of one of the common burdens that medical practitioners and their loved ones bear, extended time away from each other. As well as providing much in the way of benefit to many, medicine by its nature and throughout its course calls on all of its participants to sacrifice in the name of others. A doctor's spouse or soul mate, and children, live that reality acutely.

Prior to my leaving a consuming practice for the less hectic life of academe, our family gave up planning anything on Friday nights. I was either on call, got home too late, or was too spent from the week's work to do anything but recuperate on those evenings. Shortly after we made the switch my wife commented, elatedly, "We have our Friday nights back," as we sat down for a leisurely dinner on the porch one such evening. (See the essay, *The Comeliness of Friday Evenings on the Porch* later.)

Medical families know, too, the disappointment of treasured occurrences being diminished, or even abandoned. A surgical colleague told me that the night he was to have taken his daughter and her friends to a Dixie Chicks concert on her 13th birthday, he got caught in a coronary bypass operation that got complicated and took much longer than expected. As the disappointed adolescents waited at his house, knowing that the concert had started across town, he closed the patient's chest, accompanied him to the intensive care unit, and headed home. He arrived in time to take the girls to the second half of the concert, where they stood together, dancing, and mouthing the words to each song. The patient later wrote the child a letter explaining how grateful he was to her father for saving his life, and how sorry he was that his illness had caused her pain. It was a touching gesture; but, as my friend later related, insufficient to erase the memory of her disappointment.

Most people can relate to the disappointment of the surgeon's daughter. Many fewer know the obligations of physicians in such instances, who, while not living the medical life in isolation, have lived it longest, and its on-alert, life and death, ultimate responsibility part most personally. Only physicians know what and how much it took over years to acquire and sustain the skills that enable others to put their wellbeing in our hands. Included are memories ranging from the satisfaction felt upon achieving mastery of a treatment to those more discomfiting—like the innumerable occasions of laborious effort integral to medicine. Exhausted after being up all night as an internal medicine resident, I once phoned the hospital operator from the on-call room to ask her to wake me at 6:45 a.m. "But it's 6:30 now," she said. "I know," I answered, and fell asleep within seconds, only to rise again with her call to work the rest of the day. Included, too, is the disheartening awareness physicians have of being the one recurrently late or absent, missing out on treasured occurrences, and at times letting those who support us down. Yet, doctors understand that no matter what their level of experience, when they are on duty they are subject to *The Intern's Rule*: "When do you go home? You go home when every bit of your work is done that patients need done to make them secure."

It is the combination of the seriousness of the work, the doctor's possession of expertise, and the ultimate responsibility physicians feel for those in their care that results in benefit to patients. Paradoxically, it is that combination, too, coupled with the sheer volume of work, that tallies the personal cost physicians and their loved ones pay as they lead their lives in medicine. Too frequently, that cost is excessive, many times due to the simple reality that as exquisitely trained in biomedical knowledge and technique as doctors are by their education, they and their loved ones have little knowledge beyond assumption and trial and error of how to navigate the complex and arduous medical life. Tragically and too often, the mishandling of those complexities causes harm to self or others, like the occurrence a colleague of mine with two young children recently described when he stated that he, "consumed by medicine," had no real idea of what it took to keep a household going until he became "suddenly spouseless" by way of divorce. My own experience affirms that, while a change of course is sometimes called for, the recognition of when it is fitting may be difficult, especially for the physician. Intense effort in worthy work seems so natural that it may not be clear if it habitually crosses the threshold from being necessary to exaggerated—and then potentially harmful, to the practitioner and those at home.

Mostly, medical families endure, dedicated to each other and the work. Still, how to live the life more abundantly? I have noticed that among medical trainees, cardiology fellows—now in their mid-30's and preparing to leave school for the first time since their childhood—are the most attentive and inquisitive, both to clinical information and to things *beyond the biomedical.* Expressing a desire to finally be out on their own, almost all mention, too, a desire to avoid what has been stereotypic of previous generations of doctors: having medicine dominate even to the point of exclusion other valuable aspects of life. They often ask for advice, and when they do I recommend that they find a practice that shares their values, whatever they may be; but, that even if those values include getting rich, most of them will learn that time away from work exceeds in value the acquisition of even more money. I suggest that, just as they do with patients, they take nothing for granted about their personal relationships, know and value how things are with their loved ones, explain how things are with themselves, and appreciate that they are all in the care of each other. I tell them they should expect that as time goes on they and their loved ones will grow and change, and that they should be relentless in their efforts to assure that their family grows and changes together, not apart—and, if there are children, that the identity of the parents as a couple does not get buried in the larger realities of family and work. I offer that it is not unusual to discover what seemed to be a dream job turning into a nightmare and that they may need to consider dissociating from a practice they find harmful. "A part of wisdom," the Spanish poet Antonio Machado said, "is changing one's opinions."

Beyond the more obvious day to day struggles of our patients and ourselves, separate battles are being fought by those we love, benevolently engaged in them because of the profession to which we have been called and the way we have chosen to practice it. As affirmed in the essay, *The View From Fiesole*, medicine at its finest includes a deep appreciation for their struggles, for the goodness of their work, and for the sense of warmth that awareness of their presence brings as we finally lie down to rest, in a household of beloveds, at the end of a noble day.

————

# THE LOVELY DAY

Leaning out in piercing winds
on darkened afternoons,
when solstice souls can't comprehend
the thought of future Junes,

Or caught up in an inner storm
which blunts the noble effort made,
and dulls the sense of others' forms,
all seeming muted shades,

In press of vital burdens due—
a pause—I smiling say,
while feeling them yet sensing you,
"It's such a lovely day."[20]

-------

[20] Hergott L. The Lovely Day. *Ad Libitum, Annals of Internal Medicine.* 2016; 164:58.

# THE COMELINESS OF FRIDAY
# EVENINGS ON THE PORCH

In my 21st year of practicing cardiology I was surprisingly invited to leave the medical group and the hospital in which I worked and move to the University of Colorado School of Medicine. It took only a short period of time for me to decide that I should make the move. Though I knew I would have a considerable drop in income, I wanted to spend the last third of my career teaching medical students, residents, and cardiology fellows as well as seeing patients.

Still, the income had to be something reasonable if I were to transfer. My wife, Diane, who kept track of our finances, calculated the lowest salary we could accept and still run the household and have some savings. Our three children were in their 20's by that time and on their own, so we could live on less than we had over the previous several years. Shortly after Diane made the calculation I had a breakfast meeting with the Chief of Cardiology at the University, where he was to offer me the job and salary.

I was hoping for a salary higher than what Diane had calculated, but what the chief offered was exactly what she had calculated. Disappointed but honored to be invited to the faculty I said a grateful, "Yes."

As our family sat for dinner on our back porch a few weeks after my new job Diane strikingly said, "We have our Friday nights back."

Unsure for an instant about what she meant, I quickly knew exactly what she meant. At dinner times on Friday nights when I was in private practice I would either still be on call at the hospital, staying late to finish the week's office responsibilities, or be too tired when I got home to do anything with the family. We had our Friday nights back indeed, and as I thought about it I was overcome by a richness of joy rather than affluence.

Ten years later, our son, Zachary, who lived in Denver and was a flight instructor, died in an airplane crash of which he was not the pilot. Zach's brother and sister had moved away, so after Zach's death, Friday dinner on the porch was just Diane and me.

One Friday evening not long after Zach's death, *I* suddenly said something striking to Diane, about another benefit from my having joined the University, "I had ten years of Friday nights with Zach."

As I think about it now, another ten years having passed, I sometimes think of memories of Zach on those Friday nights—and then of his absence, and then of my missing him so.

––––––

# ON GAZING OUT THE CORNER WINDOW

I got up to fill the birdbath,
which I saw needed filling,
and now sit gazing
at the garden
out our large corner window.

The water in the bath is still,
and mirrors transfixing autumn colors—
the golden ash above,
red maples near,
a hint of blue and white sky.

I sit—
in silence, stillness, solitude—
without expectation or thought.

The water's surface ripples.

Leaves quiver.

Grey branches sway.[21]

--------

[21] Hergott L. On Gazing Out the Corner Window. *Ad Libitum, Annals of Internal Medicine.* 2016;164(6):448.

# A BENEFICENT DELAYED DEPARTURE

It had been a particularly draining week for the pulmonologist, and he was looking forward to getting home that Friday for a late dinner and a weekend with his family. The last patient he was to see before he left was an elderly man with lung masses whom he had consulted on the day before. The patient's lung biopsy early on Friday morning had been evaluated by a pathologist, who called the pulmonologist to say the findings revealed that the patient had incurable lung cancer.

Upon hearing the results the pulmonologist called the patient's primary care doctor to inform him of the diagnosis. The primary care doctor agreed that, since he knew the patient best, he should be the one to tell him of the bad news, and that he would go to see the patient early in the afternoon to do so. It was decided that the pulmonologist would then see the patient later in the afternoon to discuss how the lung cancer might be treated in an attempt to prolong his life.

When the pulmonologist arrived on the patient's hospital ward, he began to review the man's medical chart, which would describe the events of his day. As he read the chart, and then spoke with the nurses, it became clear that the patient's primary physician had not come to tell the man about his diagnosis. Sodden from a busy week of work, his family waiting at home, and he thinking he had come only to discuss how the man's treatment might proceed, the pulmonologist recognized that the burden of delivering the news, dealing with the patient's response upon hearing it, and then discussing the possible therapies had all fallen to him. He was angered that the primary physician had not seen the patient—nor let the pulmonologist know that he had not— and he felt a bit sorry for himself for having to do both his and someone else's job in a dreadful situation. He knew he would do his duty but committed to himself that he would make the visit as short as possible.

The visit at the patient's bedside began as expected, with a look of shock and despair on the man's face as the news was delivered. There was then an uncomfortably long period of silence. The physician remained silent, feeling that he had said everything there was for him to say. As the silence continued, he had the dispiriting feeling that the visit was going to take much longer than he wanted—and he could see that the course of events was largely out of his control.

The physician expected the patient to express what would be natural upon hearing such news—distress over his life ending, and fear about the illness and suffering he was destined to experience. But that was not what the patient's silence indicated, and when he finally spoke he said something the pulmonologist never forgot: "My wife," the man said softly. "Whatever will she do without me?" No tears shed for himself, no fear or trembling about what he was going to go through and then die; only concern for his beloved wife of many years.

The visit then took a radical turn, as did the attitude of the physician. He was deeply touched by what he heard and, before going into the specifics of the patient's illness and its treatment, he sat back in his chair and spent the next hour hearing the story of the couple's long life together—how they met and courted, their family life, health problems she had, and more.

After that the pulmonologist explained in detail the patient's condition and its implications, and how treatments would be planned if the patient agreed. He asked the patient if he had any questions, addressed the few he did have, and before leaving expressed his sorrow about the patient's cancer.

In spending that tender time together the pulmonologist venerated and, in a way, blessed the patient—whose sharing of the story also blessed the doctor. As he approached his car the doctor felt a sense of completion in him. He no longer felt fatigued. On the contrary, he felt he had more to give when he got home than he would have expected that night—deeply grateful for his gift to the world as a physician, and for the warm presence of his beloveds, patiently waiting at home, once more.

Nota Bene: Fortunately, the story of the patient and the pulmonologist was published decades ago, and remembered in its essence. Unfortunately, beyond the specifics of the story, neither the essay nor the author could be identified or recalled. What is written beyond the specifics is intended to honor the author and the essay.

--------

# A TENDER, COMFORTING SOMETHING

Gazing out our large corner window
after a week away
I see the birdbath empty
and rise from the chair
without thought.

Outside, a chill—
natural on the threshold of winter.
The hose feels stiff
and crackles as I lift it,
its water frozen—
I hope only in part.

The faucet fully open
produces a spray from its source,
but no water flows.

Shaking and bending the hose gently
yields the disappointing same.

Thirsty birds
will have to wait—
but only wait.
My affection for them
assures their needs met
when nature brings warmth.

Returning to the chair,
I pass by the dining room table

and am drawn to a color photo
on the newspaper's front page.

A child is being carried—
still,
limp,
dead—
by his father—
sobbing,
lost—
somewhere in a faraway land
of war.
My affection for the child and his father—
his suffering mother unseen,
his sisters and brothers,
aunts and uncles,
teachers and friends—
brings sadness,
then anger,
then helplessness.

Unlike the thirsty birds
I know of nothing I can assure
these beloveds—
hearts frozen
by a chill
this time
the unnatural has brought.

Would it comfort them to feel
there is one in the distance
who cares,
suffers with them,
would never cause them harm?

I want to bless them.

Later in the day—
the birdbath full—
four ravens come
to the branches of the ash
that shades the bath.
Two-by-two they alight
to drink
vigilantly.

I long for the arrival of the hawks,
who bless the bath—
and me—
when they come.
But they rarely come,
and always alone.

The ravens will have to do,
as I—
far away and unimagined—
will have to do.

I can soothe the thirsty birds.

I can offer a blessing to my brothers and sisters—
hoping they will feel
in the soft kiss of a gentle breeze
a tender, comforting something.[22]

– Dedicated to Thomas Friedman

--------

[22] Hergott L. A Tender, Comforting Something. *Ars Medica*, 2016;11(Issue 2): 15–18.

# MAKING IT FROM HOME TO FIRST

*Everything goes away.*

– James Finley

"You have terrible arthritis in your fingers," the orthopedist said immediately after an x-ray image of two hands appeared on his computer screen. Even as a cardiologist I could see that the distal interphalangeal joints of all the fingers were absent the cartilage seen in other joints. "Bone on bone there," he added, pointing to several places on the image. He had obtained an x-ray because I showed him a small, tender nodule on one finger that I assumed to be a Heberden node, and thus a sign of focal osteoarthritis. As I looked at the image I thought, "How could I have severe arthritis of my hands when I can swim, garden, and swing my baby granddaughter around without limitation?" I suspected that the orthopedist had mistakenly brought someone else's x-ray up on the screen. But there it was, disappointingly but convincingly visible on the image, my name.

I cannot say that seeing the findings on the x-ray has been devastating, but I haven't felt the same, or as good, since. My knowing especially that the cartilage is not coming back has imposed a sense of self disturbingly different from what I had known. There have been other incidents in the past decade signifying that something was changing about who I am, or at least what I am. Who is that guy in our family photo, for instance, and why does his face look so different from the one I see in the mirror? Why do I so often feel stiff getting out of a chair or car? Is it the statin drug I take, or something else? Why do my slacks fit more snugly in the absence of weight gained? These are not real questions, of course, since I know their answers. They are at best rhetorical and more precisely diversionary. The asking of such questions is a way to avoid ascribing true meaning to the *Whiskey, Tango, Foxtrot!* incidents to which they relate. Being only mildly disturbing, such incidents have been easy to pass by. Having seen on the x-ray what can only be described as ravaged parts of my body, though, has made it harder for my mind to turn from what is happening to me.

Aging is not a thing unfamiliar. From early in our lives we observe its changes in others. Until we reach a certain physiologic age, awareness of the effects of aging is wholly an experience of the other. Noticing such effects in oneself is of the self and can provoke concern for what other degeneration is to follow, how soon, and how much. Such awareness also brings the potential to feel less than whole, one of the definitions of suffering.

Like its frequent and even more unwelcome companion, disease, aging brings loss of various kinds—partial and complete, physical and soulful. The person affected deals with both the decrement in function and the adjustment to the decrement. Much loss associated with aging is intensely personal—mobility, sight, hearing, cognition, sexual function; and, often the deepest felt, the loss of a beloved. Other loss associated with aging is experienced indirectly, occurring to friends and loved ones but affecting the self nonetheless, no person being an island. Pondering my newly recognized bodily loss has led me to look for events past and present that might help me understand and deal with what is and what is to come.

Only one sentinel event of the past regarding aging comes to mind. Having finished my work in the early evening on my 40th birthday I somehow felt compelled to drive to a nearby convenience store, where I purchased a six-pack of beer and a pack of cigarettes. I returned to the hospital and sat in solitude in the cardiologists' lounge, drinking the beer and smoking the cigarettes, the latter something I hadn't done in nearly 20 years.

As I sat contemplatively, drinking and smoking, a sobering thought emerged about my turning 40: You're not a kid anymore. I immediately understood the rightness of the thought, and just as quickly assented. Soon after, I got up, threw the rest of the cigarettes away, placed the remaining cans of beer in the brown bag in which they came, and went home to a dinner in celebration of my birthday. The passing of time had borne me over a transforming threshold. Still, the incident was more a reflection of the passing of time than anything very personally threatening.

Now, 32 years later, having not only aged but becoming aged, I wonder what other revelatory thoughts might apply. Thoughts that have come so far are mainly questions based on a principle that at this point in my life does imply threat, *everything goes away*: With whatever time I have left, how do I want to go out? How can I continue to be of service? How can I know when it is time to reduce my level of service and leave medicine, which has dominated my life since I was 15? To whom, and for whom, am I most responsible now? How would I like to be remembered? And, the most relevant, who do I want to be as whatever is to come comes?

A few answers to the questions have surfaced, occasionally in the negative. I do not want to be like the elderly physician I came upon as he stood in a restaurant line waiting to pay his bill while leaning on a cane. When asked how he was doing in retirement, he mentioned an arthritic condition he had acquired. "It's bad enough going from being somebody to being nobody," he said bitterly. "But it's awful being nobody with a disability." His sense of self-worth seemed to be largely related to his identity of being, not having been, a physician.

Regarding the question of when to leave medicine, I know the time will come to step aside, but I also have a sense of how difficult it might be to walk away from the richly consuming life of medical practice. I do not want to be like physicians I have known who held on beyond the point when they were of real benefit to their patients. Some stayed so long they were a burden to their patients—and a few to the point where their presence, or absence, didn't matter. A common theme to overstaying seemed to emanate from the physicians having recognized that, although the hard-earned title Doctor remains, self-identity changes in the absence of patients to care for.

Insight about staying or leaving has come from an unlikely source, the story of a friend of mine, former All-Pro National Football League lineman Ed White. Reconsidering his retirement from football, Ed White had a sentinel event that made him decide: he hurt his leg trying to run out a ground ball in a family softball game. He stayed retired, stating, "If you can't make it from home to first in a family softball game you can't play in the NFL."

What might such sentinel events be for aging physicians, indicating that we cannot or should not continue in medicine? Will we recognize which events are sentinel and which are incidental? Who decides? How much of a struggle to continue is appropriate, or honorable? We will be remembered in part by how we handle our leaving. Symbolically relevant for us might be Warren Buffett's warning that it can take 20 years to build a reputation, and 5 minutes to ruin it.

The most powerful thought that has come since I saw the image of my hands on the computer screen has not been in the form of a question but of a second threatening principle: *You're not going to get away with this much longer*. This in my case means being at an excessive and unhealthy body weight. Not getting away with it refers to the likelihood of developing in the near future at least one of the conditions being in such a state can bring: more and more-limiting arthritis, diabetes, atherosclerotic events. Others' *this* could be a lifestyle that involves smoking, excess alcohol use, injurious stress, or neglect of relationships. Each condition has its potential sequelae, and the appearance of the sequelae often marks our having been borne across another important threshold, from aging to disease.

For me and others of a similar age, the clock is not only ticking but winding down. Recognizing this has brought a sense of urgency for me to abandon long-held but potentially destructive habits and to live the fullest and longest life possible—the motivation to make the required changes coming largely from a deepening sense that the people to whom I am most responsible now, and care most about, are those who love me and want me with them. I want to be with them. The balanced life I have tried to live during my career, ascribing importance to both medicine and family, is shifting in my mind toward a strong emphasis on the personal rather than professional.

The title of this essay might just as well have been "The Aged Struggle to Make It From Home to First," which can be interpreted in two ways. Because of the limitations the passing of time commonly imposes, the aged do struggle to live a functional life—to make it from home to first and beyond. And that effort is shared with those over the ages who tried to do the same. Still, the struggle for each has always been individual. How things proceed for me will substantially depend on how I respond to what I have seen—in my hands, in my head, and in my heart. Time will pass. Time will tell. But little else is assured, including time itself.

One thing of which I am certain is that, while enduring whatever degeneration and disease are to come, until I go away I will do my utmost to remain faithful to a pledge I have made each day since experiencing one of the deepest kinds of loss, that of a child, ten years ago. The pledge emanates from something found in the late Irish poet and philosopher John O'Donohue's poem, "On the Death of the Beloved"—a declaration offering a way of being that might provide sustenance to any life of struggle, which means to every life:

> *To enter each day with a generous heart.*
> *To serve the call of courage and love.*

– For Amy, Ed, and Joann White[23]

--------

[23] Hergott L. Making It From Home to First. *JAMA*. July 18, 2012.

# SOME YEARS HAVING PASSED SINCE I LOST YOU

Now,
some years having passed since I lost you,
I am sometimes bothered
that you are less often on my mind.

But, like today,
the infrequent times I am alone
with nothing to do
that familiar surge of sadness rises
to overwhelm me.

I do not fall to the floor,
trembling,
as I did in the early months.
I stand,
hand to my forehead—
I wail,
I bend,
my fingernails dig deep into my skin,
and I weep,
and weep,
and weep.

I do not write of my sudden sorrow
to let you know,

or reassure you,
that I have not forgotten us.

You know.

I write,
missing you,
tears still flowing,
grateful to be reassured myself.[24]

-------

[24] Hergott L. Some Years Having Passed Since I Lost You. *Ad Libitum, Annals of Internal Medicine*. 2018;168(6):451.

# ASPECTS OF ENDING
# A LIFELONG DREAM

As the time approached to empty my office and end a long career in the practice of cardiology I decided to take home each day one boxful of artifacts I had placed there over the years. Replete with sentiment by nature I was surprised that, day after day, I had no emotional response to removing and packing the items. Each had been "chosen for its meaning or its beauty," and each is dear to me. The artifacts signify formative and sustaining occurrences in my life that took me from the uncarved block I was at the beginning of my career to the doctor and person I am.

I gently wrapped and packed a bobble head doll of the Denver Broncos mascot, *The Barrel Man*, autographed and presented to me in gratitude by the man himself. With care I packed a desktop statue of Rodin's, *The Kiss*, which had graced every desk I had since 1979, reminding me on even the hardest workdays of the loving presence awaiting me at home. I took down without feeling a large framed photograph of Thomas Merton sitting on a rock in a field at Gethsemani Abbey, gazing at me as he rested from work there. I had hung the photo across from my desk so I would see it every day, and take inspiration from Merton's presence. It wasn't until about the fifth day, when I placed my 35-year-old stethoscope in a box, that tears came.

Why then? I think tears came because, of all the artifacts I handled, the stethoscope was most symbolic of the connection I had made with the thousands of people to whom most of my adult life was dedicated. For a long period in my early career that dedication was driven by a sense of ineptitude, and my not wanting to harm. At the end of my career, my dedication was accompanied by the gratifying feeling that I could help patients and their loved ones from the wellspring of even the most minute and remote elements of my medical being. Pondering my emotion over packing the stethoscope I realized that I was letting go of much more than what went into the boxes—and especially letting go of patients and their loved ones, whom I would see, speak to, touch, and help no more; and whom I would miss, in the "Tender agony of parting" Jelaluddin Rumi described.

Ending a medical practice involves leaving an incalculable variety of meaningful things. I will miss the dedication, friendship, and support of colleagues, students, nurses, clinic and hospital staff, and medical administrators. I will miss hospital hallways, patient rooms, conference rooms, and what takes place in communal workplaces on hospital wards. I will miss echocardiographic, angiographic, and other images on screens revealing fascinating realities. I will miss reassuring patients and their loved ones when no disease process is found, helping to eradicate their maladies if some are found, or journeying with them if no successful treatment is available. I will miss spending my days healing.

Deeply missed will be the never-ending fascination that accompanies medical practice—as described earlier in *Playing the Moonlight Sonata From Memory*. The ongoing presence of such awesomeness around us is one of the most sustaining and fulfilling elements of doctoring.

A particularly treasured entity absent will be the sharing of humor that accompanies medical practice, and helps sustain and even guide us. On many occasions I have mentioned to medical students and young physicians that, though we are committed to compassionate care of patients, there are times when that commitment is strained, and that it is all right to feel so. We occasionally see patients who simply behave badly, and whom we may not like. I shared that in my case I have occasionally thought toward the end of such interactions I would like to say to the patient, "Come back to see me in forty-six weeks." "What was that, doctor?" "Come back to see me in four-to-six weeks." (With patients who behave especially badly, the fantasy of saying "sixty-eight weeks" feels even better.)

Medical humor can educate us about ourselves. My nephew, an excellent emergency medicine physician, humbly shared a story that took place early in his career that demonstrates opportunities medicine offers to sometimes take ourselves less seriously. A construction worker had fallen from the second floor of a building onto a long, exposed segment of rebar fixed in concrete. The rebar entered his neck on one side and came out just below his eye on the other. Workers quickly sawed the segment of rebar from the concrete and sent the man off in an ambulance with the penetrating rebar in place.

When the patient arrived in the emergency department, my nephew, in an attempt to determine if there was any damage beyond the obvious from the fall asked, "Where does it hurt?" The patient, his head still, with an expression of *negative awe* on his face, directed his eyes toward the questioner, paused, and with his hand pointed to the rebar entering his neck.

And last, just after my finishing a lecture some years ago, a young man from the audience approached and introduced himself. He was an internist in my large medical group. He thanked me for the lecture, and then added, "You and I have a common patient I just met," and mentioned the patient's name.

"Oh, good," I said, and continued, "Do you know that he is a member of the world renowned Takacs String Quartet?" "Yes," he said, "they are Hungarians."

"Do you know the story of how they came to America?" I asked.

"No," he responded curiously.

Being a friend of the quartet members I then shared some of their history. I explained that even as young men they were very successful, and frequently toured in Europe. I mentioned that when they toured out of Hungary, to keep them from escaping to another country, the communist government would not allow them to bring their families with them.

On one occasion, though, for reasons unclear, after the quartet had played many concerts out of Hungary with no political complications, the government allowed them to take their wives and children along.

The four musicians and their wives and children packed their bags, left the country, and never came back. They left their parents, brothers and sisters, friends, teachers, homes, and native country.

The young physician was amazed by the story.

"Wow," he said. "I had no idea they all defecated together."

Hearing him say the word 'defecate' rather than 'defect,' my initial response—vividly remembered still—was to keep from forming in my mind a vision of the scene he had just described.

I was successful in suppressing the disturbing image, but I felt the need to respond, yet not embarrass or correct my young colleague.

"Yes," I said, "they all left together," and we parted.

Some things left behind will not be missed. I will not miss carrying out a self-imposed penance on each of the 1000 echocardiograms I read every year because I failed to make a diagnosis during my first year in practice 37 years ago. A patient had been admitted to the hospital by his internist for very mild and fleeting chest discomfort. I wondered why the patient had been admitted for such mild symptoms, and found no cardiovascular cause for his discomfort the evening I consulted on him. His doctor then arranged an upper endoscopy for the next morning. During the endoscopy the patient died. Upon receiving a phone call at home from the gastroenterologist informing me of the death I drove to the hospital that Saturday morning to console him for losing a patient during a procedure, presumably from an anesthesia accident. When I arrived, the patient's body was still on the examination table. That afternoon, an autopsy showed that he died of an ascending aortic dissection with sudden and lethal pericardial tamponade during the procedure.

Transthoracic echocardiography has a low sensitivity for diagnosing ascending aortic dissections. The patient never even had an echocardiogram. But, as a young clinician, the vision of seeing my patient dead on the table, knowing I had failed to make a threatening cardiovascular diagnosis, made me pledge without thought to never miss another aortic dissection. Thus, I have spent an inordinate amount of time looking over, and over, the four or so images that show the aorta on a standard echocardiogram. As I do so I know I am being overly cautious, but I do it anyway, continuing to find unsatisfying the harsh but well-intended and sage comment of a senior internist at my hospital after the event, "You'll probably miss the next one, too. These things present in very occult ways."

There are some things about medicine I will not only not miss but would like to see changed. The most disturbing of these is the devolution of medical practice, powered by outside forces driven by economics and profit, to the point where the *soul of medicine* is threatened. As time constraints in patient-doctor interactions and other pressures worsen, clinicians—who have nothing to prove regarding expertise, diligence, dedication, and effort—are expected to prove their worth in ways peripheral to patient care that have somehow become central. The worst of these are expectations that make real something Thomas Merton warned us about 50 years ago, becoming "A mere utensil for production."

A recent statement by a dedicated clinical psychologist considering early retirement clarified for me substantial reasons why medical practitioners may feel stressed. In explaining why she was considering retiring she said, "I don't have compassion fatigue, which is known in my field. I have responsibility fatigue." The conflict and frustration felt practicing medicine by a system's way of doing things rather than our own can make clinicians susceptible to both. Following now from a distance, I am hoping that enlightenment—in the name of patients, practitioners, and our culture—will prevail, and lead to positive, sustainable change.

My dream of being a doctor began when I was 15 years old. I am now 70 years old, and experiencing aspects of ending that lifelong dream. These are aspects of *a* lifelong dream, specific to medicine, not *the* lifelong dream desired by every person: a lengthy, fulfilling, and evolutionary life, spent longing to love and be loved. My lifelong dream has transitioned into *the* lifelong dream—which, of course, was my foundation the entire time.

At a dinner party recently, I asked the question, "If you could live your life again, not knowing in doing so how it would progress, but living each day as it had happened, and you had the choice to live it again or not, what would you choose?" It was such a bizarre, jarring, "Does this guy need help?" question that no one had an answer.

I have an answer. Early in my thinking, because of a painfully remembered childhood and the often-brutal experiences of medical training and practice in the early years, the answer was No. With considerably more thought, and taking Thomas Merton's advice to "see life in its wholeness," as I reflected on my life—including what is to come—the answer became an absolute Yes.

**Postscript:**

When friends ask how I am doing in retirement I share with them that I am "having a blast." My days are full but not hectic, and sated with meaning and joy.

Shortly after leaving my practice I began to occasionally see outpatients for a large cardiology group that had an access problem. My schedule is structured so that I do consultative work only—seeing patients once and then sending them back to their primary care providers or to other cardiologists in the group if follow up is needed.

Contrary to the practice I left, the job is temporary, I have no office, I barely get to know the patients, and when I walk through the hallways of the large medical building I work in approximately no one knows who I am.

I read a handful of echocardiograms on the day I work. Knowing why, and knowing better, I still spend an inordinate amount of time on the aortic images. I am not quite free—thankfully, in a way.

––––––––

**Post-postscript:**

As with *Aspects of Ending a Lifelong Dream,* when one of my essays gets published I typically receive around 200 e-mails, cards, or other communications from readers around the world. In one e-mail responding to this essay an internist in Monterey, Mexico wrote to thank me for writing the essay. I responded with thanks to him. I was surprised to receive another message from him. This time, the internist had a question about the intensity of my echo reading. "The story of the patient who died from an ascending aortic dissection is powerful," he wrote. "I think things like this affect all doctors, and we have to live with it, with a heavy burden on our shoulders." Then came a sage question: "I am curious. May I ask, how many aortic dissections did you find in your exhaustive searches?"

I was stunned by his question—immediately knowing not only the answer but also the implication of the answer being an epiphany for me. I responded to his e-mail, thanking him for asking the deeply relevant question, and wrote that I had detected "exactly zero" occult aortic dissections through my diligence. I had never asked myself the question he did, probably by being blinded by guilt and thus unaware that all the time, effort, and stress I spent on such interpretations had made no difference to any patient over almost four decades. I could certainly be accused of a lack of insight about the value of my extra effort over those years but making the commitment I did standing next to my patient's dead body resulted in a punitive sentence of prolonged meticulousness rather than insight.

I did diagnose some aortic dissections on echocardiograms over that period of time—even a few that other readers had missed. But the aortic tears on those studies, while perhaps not obvious, were also not occult to an experienced reader.

After the interaction with my Mexican colleague I read a few more echocardiograms in the same way I had for all those years. As I did I could feel the futility of doing so and did something I never thought I would do. I stopped obsessing about the echocardiograms—and finally accepted without reservation or negotiation the responsibility of missing the diagnosis that led to the patient's death so long ago.[25]

———

[25] Hergott L. Aspects of Ending a Lifelong Dream. *JAMA*. 2017;317(2):137–138.

# DECLARATION OF FAITH

I believe in
The Power of Love,
Democracy,
and
Science—
in that order.[26]

-------

[26] Hergott L. Declaration of Faith. *Ad Libitum, Annals of Internal Medicine.* 2017;167(6):435.

# A CONCEIVABLE POINT
# OF DEPARTURE

*We shall not cease from exploration, and the end of all our exploring will be to arrive where we started and know the place for the first time.*

– T.S. Eliot

*To know when to stop
To know when you can go no further
By your own action,
This is the right beginning.*

– Chuang Tzu

In my last week as a part time cardiologist two years after my full time practice I was scheduled to work in an outpatient clinic for three days. The appointment slots for those days were filled. There were several of my patients, though, who were not scheduled but had ongoing tests and questions that needed attention. I felt it would be best for the patients to get their concerns and conditions taken care of before I left the practice, so they wouldn't have to wait for weeks to get them addressed by a new cardiologist. Taking care of the patients' issues up front would also make things easier for the doctors they would eventually see. My nurse and I agreed to add appointments at the end of some already-filled schedules that week, and see a few patients on a day off. The last patient we saw that week, and thus in my career, was challenging.

The patient had agreed to come in late one afternoon, after all the other patients were seen. As the time approached for us to see her the nurse and I noticed that the patient's name was not on the computer list showing that she had checked in. As I took care of some other details, I scanned the check-in list every 15 minutes. When all of the other work was done, 30 minutes after her scheduled appointment, her name was still not on the list. She wasn't coming.

Just before leaving for the afternoon, the nurse called the patient, who said she forgot that her appointment was that day. We then scheduled her for a 10:00 a.m. appointment the next day, which was an off day, but one on which we had already agreed to see another patient earlier. The patient who missed her appointment on the first day did so again on the second day. I found her absence annoying, since we had gone out of our way to help her, but the nurse and I agreed to try one more time to get the patient into clinic. We offered her an appointment the next and final day, another off-day for us. Before the nurse hung up after arranging the third visit, she had the patient verbalize her understanding by repeating, 'My appointment is at 9:00 a.m. tomorrow morning.'

On the final day, with no other patient scheduled, we waited for her to check in, but her name did not appear on the list at 9:00 o'clock, 9:30, or 9:45. At 10:00 a.m., just as I was finishing the last few things that needed to be done before I left for good, the patient's name appeared on the check-in list. She had finally arrived, and my annoyance surfaced again—but just for a moment. A thought suddenly came to me about why she might have missed her appointments—a thought that implied something far more disturbing than her being late. Having seen her as a patient intermittently over a number of years, I remembered her as being friendly and thoughtful. As soon as I asked myself the question, 'Why is she causing so much trouble?', I was afraid that I knew the answer.

As I entered the examination room where the patient and her husband sat I welcomed them, and in a pleasantly puzzled tone said that we were expecting to see her at 9:00 a.m. She said she thought her appointment was at 10:00 a.m.—the time of her previous day's appointment. Her response increased my concern, not about any cardiovascular issues but from something much more in her case, which prompted me to ask a question I would rather not have to ask, 'I haven't seen you in a while. How is your memory?'

'Oh, I have always been a bit scrambled with details,' she cheerfully said. Her husband objected forcefully, as he briskly leaned forward in his chair and definitively said, 'Her memory is bad, and it's getting worse'—which confirmed my suspicion about why she had missed her appointments. She had forgotten the details of her visit. Her memory was probably worsening, and needed attention. Her cognitive problem could have been as relatively benign as a subdural hematoma—a collection of blood on the surface of her brain, acquired when she would have bumped her head sometime—to the early stages of a cognitive impairment such as Alzheimer's Disease. I expressed my concern over her memory issues, and recommended that she see her primary care doctor to further define and treat them.

We proceeded with her visit, took care of her cardiac issues, and I asked her husband to contact her primary care doctor to initiate testing. I said goodbye to both, wished them well, and sent off a note to her primary care doctor about my concerns, to make certain she would be called to come in and be evaluated.

———————

After the patient left I sat restfully in my office chair, realizing that in treating my patient I had symbolically come full circle in my long career. My patient had a neurologic problem rather than a cardiac problem. She needed a primary care doctor—like I had been for the years prior to my cardiology training. The visit was also a classic example of why clinicians should not be judgmental, not in a hurry, and always aware of the possibility that patients may have issues beyond what they come in for. More than just her cardiology status was addressed during the visit. The patient was treated with respect, and not chastised for her absences. She was treated comprehensively and compassionately by everyone who saw her that day—their feeling, as always, that caring for patients is a *privilege*, not a burden.

As I looked around the office I noticed that the few photographs I had placed there were in a cardboard box, that there were no documents on my desk to address, no electrocardiograms or echocardiograms to read, no phone calls to make, and nothing on my computer to take care of. What came to me as I sat was the vivid image of the day I decided to commit myself to being a doctor at the age of 15, and the equally vivid awareness that when I walked away on that final day, at the age of 72, I would be a doctor no more. The things I had so very arduously learned and applied in pre-medical years, medical school, internship, residency, cardiology fellowship, and extensive cardiology practice would be of little use to anyone. I knew there would be other satisfying experiences in my life—but likely none to match, or be so privileged by, my life in medicine.

Finally, I got up, left my office, said goodbye to the nurses and clinic staff, took the elevator down, alone, to the lobby, and walked away—eternally grateful for a life in medicine, and for the presence of *the soul of medicine* that so often accompanied me.

------

# DEVOTION IN A TIME OF MOURNING

*Forlornly aware of the mantles we bear*
*in various states of duress,*
*my heart warmly bounds*
*as I see all around*
*our silent pronouncement of,*
*"Yes."*

While we work and hope for the better we give ourselves as abundantly as possible for the needs of a patient.

------

# REGARDING THE FRONT COVER

The photo of the lotus pond was taken in a garden at the Heian Palace in Kyoto, Japan. The evolvement of the lotus flower, from its beginning in mud to its rising to the top of the pond, and being beautiful, represents the evolution of medical care to come—from our so often being in symbolic 'mud,' to the flowering of the soul of medicine.

CPSIA information can be obtained
at www.ICGtesting.com
Printed in the USA
BVHW040816250720
584567BV00001B/3